Primary Care and Social Services: Developing New Partnerships for Older People

National Primary Care Research and Development Series

Primary Care and Social Services: Developing New Partnerships for Older People

National Primary Care Research and Development Series

Kirstein Rummery
Caroline Glendinning

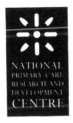

RADCLIFFE MEDICAL PRESS

Radcliffe Medical Press Ltd
18 Marcham Road, Abingdon, Oxon OX14 1AA, UK

British Library Cataloguing in Publication Data

A catalogue record for this book is available from the British Library.

ISBN 1 85775 466 2

Typeset by Advance Typesetting Ltd, Oxon
Printed and bound by TJ International Ltd, Padstow, Cornwall

The National Primary Care Research and Development Centre is a Department of Health-funded initiative, based at the University of Manchester. The NPCRDC is a multi-disciplinary centre which aims to promote high-quality and cost-effective primary care by delivering high-quality research, disseminating research findings and promoting service development, based upon sound evidence. The Centre has staff based at three collaborating sites: The National Centre at the University of Manchester, the Institute for Public Health Research and Policy at the University of Salford and the Centre for Health Economics at the University of York.

For further information about the centre, or for a copy of our research prospectus please contact

Communications Office, NPCRDC
The University of Manchester
5th Floor, Williamson Building
Oxford Road
Manchester M13 9PL

Tel: 0161 275 7126/7633
Fax: 0161 275 7600
www.npcrdc.man.ac.uk

Contents

About the authors

Kirstein Rummery is Research Fellow at the National Primary Care Research and Development Centre, University of Manchester.

Caroline Glendinning is Reader in Social Policy at the National Primary Care Research and Development Centre, University of Manchester.

Abbreviations

DH	Department of Health
HImP	health improvement programme
HMO	health management organisation
GMS	general medical services
IM&T	information management and technology
NHSE	National Health Service Executive
PASS	practice agreement with social services
PCT	primary care trust
PCG	primary care group
PHCT	primary healthcare team
PMS	personal medical services
SSD	social services department
TPP	total purchasing pilot project

1

Partnerships between primary health and social care

INTRODUCTION

British health policy during the 1990s has emphasised the key role of primary- and community-based health services in achieving major strategic changes throughout the NHS. The implementation in 1993 of the 1990 NHS and Community Care Act gave local authority social services departments lead responsibility for planning and purchasing domiciliary, residential and nursing home care services. Yet despite the lead roles now assigned to both these service sectors, difficulties in achieving closer working between them remain. Primary health and social services are therefore at risk of:

- an absence of co-ordination and coherence
- being financially inefficient, and
- being ineffective in achieving their objectives.

For patients, service users and their families the consequences all too often include fragmentation, lack of continuity, delay and difficulties in finding out what is available, from whom and (when social care services are involved) at what cost.

Current policy changes which promote opportunities for closer working relationships between primary and community health and social services offer some opportunities to address these issues. Two main policy developments are of interest.

The December 1997 White Paper for England, *The New NHS: modern, dependable*[1] and the subsequent 1999 NHS Act require NHS organisations at all levels to collaborate both with each other and with other statutory services. The third of six 'key principles' in *The New NHS* is 'to get the NHS to work in *partnership*. By breaking down organisational barriers and forging stronger links with local authorities, the needs of the patient will be put at the centre of the care process'.[1] One concrete example of this is the duty to have social services representation on primary care group (PCG) boards.

A consultative document *Partnership in Action*[2] outlines three options designed to facilitate partnerships between the NHS and local authorities:

- pooled budgets
- delegating to a lead commissioning agency, and
- integrated provider organisations.

The necessary legislative changes are also included in the 1999 NHS Act. The first new *Partnership in Action* schemes are expected to go 'live' from April 2000, at the same time as the first new primary care trusts (PCTs).

This book aims to assist health and social care organisations and professionals to develop new ways of working together, in order to deliver more effective and efficient services to older people with complex needs. It draws on a range of research to help managers and practitioners on both sides of the primary/community health and social care divide make the most of these new opportunities. While joint planning and joint commissioning between health and local authorities has a long and well-evaluated history,[3] the involvement of primary and community health services alongside (or instead of) health authorities in planning and purchasing services with local authority social services has been far less common. Chapter 2 of this book reviews these latter experiences, as they will be particularly relevant for the activities of the new English primary care groups.

The experience of locating social services staff in primary and community health services settings in order to achieve closer day-to-day working relationships is much more common. Chapter 3 reviews the available evidence on the organisation, management and effectiveness of these partnerships between frontline professionals.

The movement for evidence-based medicine in the NHS is creating expectations that developments in areas of policy and practice not confined to clinical practice should be similarly grounded in firm research evidence. There is, therefore, a need to monitor and evaluate service partnerships, to ensure that objectives are being met in services for older people. However, this can be complex; for example, the costs and benefits of new service partnerships for frontline staff, for service managers, for service users and for informal carers may all differ from each other. Chapter 4 therefore suggests strategies for evaluating new frontline collaborative arrangements, with a particular emphasis on approaches which can be incorporated into routine service monitoring and audit.

Finally, Chapter 5 takes a speculative look into the future. The major changes in the organisation and funding of NHS and local authority services which are currently being introduced could radically alter the structures and boundaries of these services in the future. What lessons can be learned which might help redraw the health and social services map for the future?

Many of the joint commissioning initiatives and the frontline collaboration projects have been reviewed and evaluated. However, these reviews and evaluations have tended to be published in academic books and journals, or as commissioned reports with limited local circulation; neither source is easily accessible to busy managers and practitioners. This book therefore draws on a wide range of published and 'grey' material; each chapter concludes with a summary of key points.

THE PROBLEM OF THE HEALTH/SOCIAL CARE DIVIDE

Since the post-war welfare state was established in Britain, the boundaries between health and local authority services have been problematic for health professionals, social workers, managers and service users alike. Different statutory responsibilities, organisational barriers, funding streams and professional cultures have combined to impede both the joint planning and the frontline co-ordination of services. Since the mid-1970s, resource constraints have added to the tightening of boundaries around the core responsibilities of statutory services, with less and less scope for investment and flexibility at the margins. As each agency has narrowed its focus in response to these pressures, the risk has increased that people with complex health and social care needs fall between the responsibilities of different services and professionals.

During the 1980s, collaboration between health and social services around services for older people occurred largely through joint consultative committees and joint care planning teams. These involved senior officers from relevant health and social services authorities (the latter sometimes devolved down to area or divisional levels), along with representatives of key voluntary sector organisations. While some areas achieved agreement in principle to joint strategies for older people, for the most part health and local authorities remained hostile to each other and there were wide gaps between strategic agreements and service delivery.[4] Primary and community health services were rarely involved to any significant degree in joint planning.

During the early 1990s, joint planning was replaced by joint commissioning,[5] which placed greater emphasis on assessing the needs of the population and translating strategic plans into effective use of resources to develop services. Again, this largely involved health authorities working with social services managers, rather than primary and community health services. However, a combination of recent policy changes has created major imperatives on primary and community health staff to take an active role in developing closer partnerships, at all levels, with their local authority counterparts.

First, the concept of a 'primary care-led NHS'[6] emphasised the role of GPs in commissioning and purchasing medical and nursing services on behalf of their patients. It also enhanced the role of primary and community health services in providing treatments for patients who might previously have been referred to hospital.

> *With primary care-led purchasing reinforcing a strategic shift in the pattern and configuration of acute services, the traditional role of the hospital is likely to be provided in primary care and intermediate settings.*[7]

The commissioning role of GPs was eventually extended beyond the voluntary (and allegedly divisive) fundholding and locality commissioning schemes to all GPs, through the establishment in April 1999 of primary care groups.[1]

On the local authority side, the 1993 community care changes gave social services departments lead responsibility for assessing the needs of older and disabled people and for funding appropriate domiciliary, residential and nursing home services. GPs and other primary health workers wanting to avoid hospital admission or expedite the discharge of patients who have difficulty living independently in the community therefore now have to negotiate the 'gatekeeping' role of local authority social services departments. The community care changes also assumed that GPs and other primary and community health professionals would contribute to multi-disciplinary community care assessments.[8]

However, for much of the 1990s, developments in both the NHS and local government did not provide fertile ground for the development of closer partnerships.

- Major structural changes took place in both the NHS – the creation and subsequent abolition of market-type relationships between health purchasing and providing organisations; and in local government – a rolling programme of local government reform[9] and the development of external markets of voluntary and for-profit provider organisations. Because these changes involved the introduction of competition in the commissioning of services, they were inimical to the development of partnerships in which trust and a familiarity with the broader organisational contexts and priorities of other partners are important success factors.

- Neither local government reorganisation, the changes following the introduction of the NHS internal market in the early 1990s, nor the recent creation of PCGs have aimed to achieve alignment of the boundaries between English health and local authorities. Moreover, the problems of aligning boundaries are increased by the key role assigned to GPs in commissioning and purchasing services. Whereas health authorities may be able to align their boundaries on a geographical basis, GPs commission services for patients within the catchment areas of their unevenly distributed practices. Under the internal market, therefore, local authority social services departments had to liaise with a potentially large number of different GP purchasers and commissioners within their boundaries. With the formation of PCGs the overall number of primary care partners has been reduced but problems of defining common boundaries and eligible populations remain.

- GPs, whose perspectives are likely to dominate PCGs, have also tended traditionally to focus on the needs of individual patients or groups of patients registered with their practices.[10] Aggregate information, even at the level of GP practice populations, and the systematic use of that information by GPs to inform decision making and planning has traditionally been poor.[11] The involvement of primary health service users in setting service priorities and objectives has also been under-developed.[11,12] In contrast, local authorities have long adopted a population-based approach to needs assessment and service planning. Since 1992, they have been required regularly to assess the needs of their local populations for community care services and review the appropriateness of existing services. Consultation with users has been a mandatory element of this process.[13]

* Although the various fundholding and commissioning experiments gave many GPs experience of planning and purchasing services, they did so through conferring *purchasing power*, not encouraging collaboration and joint working. Those GPs in total purchasing pilot projects, for example, who expressed interest in purchasing continuing and community care services showed little evidence of collaboration with their local social services departments.[12]

THE NEW EMPHASIS ON PARTNERSHIP IN POLICY AND PRACTICE

Both the NHS and local authorities have, since 1997, experienced growing pressures and incentives to work in closer partnership. This emphasis on partnership follows directly from the recognition that ill health and health inequalities are caused by factors which lie largely outside the remit of the NHS, such as social and economic circumstances, environmental and lifestyle factors and the accessibility of services like education, transport and leisure.[14]

The Government recognises the complex causes of ill health and the part that economic and social factors have to play.[15]

Local health improvement plans (HImPs) provide a strategic framework for investment and service development, which are intended to shape the priorities and activities of local authorities as much as those of health services purchasers and providers.[1] Similarly, the objectives which have been set for health action zones include improving joint working between the NHS and local government, so that resources, goals and objectives are equally shared.[16]

Unlike earlier joint planning and joint commissioning activities, primary and community health services are now expected to be at the centre of these developments. Rather like the lettering running through a stick of rock, *The New NHS: modern, dependable* stresses the importance of partnerships at all levels of NHS and local authority relationships. Primary care groups are required to include social services representatives, as well as community health service providers, on their governing bodies. Health authorities and NHS trusts are also required to work in partnership alongside local authorities. NHS regional offices and the Department of Health's Social Services Inspectorate will jointly monitor indicators of partnership activities across health and social services organisations.

USERS' AND PATIENTS' EXPERIENCES OF THE HEALTH/SOCIAL CARE DIVIDE

The separation between NHS and local authority services is particularly problematic for people with mental health problems, disabilities, frail older people and families and children who are at risk or need extra support. The boundaries between these services are further underlined, from the point of view of users, by the common practice of charging for local authority social services,[17,18] in contrast to NHS services which remain free at the point of use. Thus the boundaries between day, respite or domiciliary services which are provided for 'health' reasons and those which are provided for 'social' reasons can have major financial implications for users.

There have already been significant steps in a few parts of England to integrate community-based clinical, nursing and social work support for people with mental health problems through the establishment of integrated mental health and social care trusts and community mental health teams.[19,20] However, primary health services, in either their commissioning or provider roles, appear to be marginal to these developments. There are fewer reports of initiatives which integrate health and social work services for families and children who are experiencing problems. However, a small number of pioneering pilot projects suggest there may be considerable potential for improving the liaison between primary healthcare teams and social services departments to provide better services for vulnerable children and families.[21,22]

There are, however, major pressures to improve collaboration between primary and community health and social services in relation to frail older people, particularly those who are at risk of being admitted to hospital or residential care.

- Older people (and particularly the very elderly) constitute a growing proportion of the population. By 2011, well over a million people will be aged 85 and over[23] and at increased risk of experiencing long-term health and other care problems. A high proportion will be living alone and therefore more likely to be relying on formal health and social services rather than friends and relatives to provide care and support.
- There are continuing imperatives to reduce the numbers of hospital admissions for non-medical reasons and cut length of stay for those who are admitted because of acute illness or surgery. A high proportion of such admissions are of older people. These imperatives have in turn created very considerable pressures on both primary health and local authority social services to find alternative ways of supporting and caring for frail older people in the community, instead of admitting them to hospital.

It has been argued that services for frail older people are now a prime focus of developments in health and welfare services in most advanced industrial societies, because 'welfare systems change first at points of pressure where established policies and solutions are no longer working or cannot be sustained'.[24] Many of the joint commissioning and frontline partnerships which have involved primary and community health services working alongside social services have focused on improving the appropriateness and co-ordination of services for frail older people. This book draws on these experiences and, if the previous analysis is correct, they will show the way for more widespread changes.

IMPLEMENTING PARTNERSHIPS BETWEEN NHS AND LOCAL AUTHORITY SERVICES

A series of associated legislative, policy and managerial initiatives have been announced which are designed to transform the rhetoric of partnership into reality. Additional resources, released by the Government's Comprehensive Spending Review, have also been made available to support partnership developments.

- From 1998, local authorities and health authorities have been required to develop joint investment plans, working together to review, plan and commission long-term care, rehabilitation and recovery services for frail older and disabled people.[25] This marks a distinct change from former policies which encouraged the clear demarcation of service responsibilities and boundaries, which had been implicit in earlier measures such as local continuing care agreements on the limits of respective NHS and social services responsibilities. Joint in-vestment plans are also required to clarify arrangements for multi-disciplinary assessments of older people's health and social care needs.

- In 1998, the Department of Health issued a single set of guidelines on the service development priorities for the NHS and local authority social services. In addition to their individual responsibilities, both organisations must take a shared lead in tackling health inequalities, improving mental health services and improving the independence of disabled and older people and carers; 'because health and social care in these areas are inextricably linked, both organisations have a major contribution to make and both regard them as priorities ... in almost all areas, health and social services have contributions to make to each other's activities.'[15] Regional offices of the NHSE are now required to collect information on a number of key 'partnership' activities and the performance management and inspection of other NHS and local authority services will be increasingly closely aligned.[15]

- The White Paper on local authority social services[15] announced a number of new grants to be spent up to 2002. The Partnership Grant is specifically earmarked to support local authorities in developing new services in collaboration with health partners, particularly services which are able to improve rehabilitation opportunities, avoid unnecessary hospital admissions and respond to seasonal demands for extra health and other services. The special Prevention Grant is intended to be used, again in collaboration with health purchasers and providers, on non-intensive community care services to reduce risk and promote independence among older and disabled people.

- From April 2000, opportunities for closer integration of health and local authority services will be possible through the use of pooled budgets, designated lead commissioning arrangements and integrated provider organisations.[2] In line with these proposals, the 1999 NHS Act contains permissive provision for funding streams and other statutory responsibilities to be transferred between health and local authority organisations. From April 2000, PCGs will therefore be able to apply for approval to pool budgets with, or delegate functions to, local authorities (or vice versa) and primary care trusts (PCTs) will be able to provide a range of social as well as healthcare services (and vice versa). Use of these flexibilities will initially be subject to approval by the Secretary of State.

Of course significant obstacles to closer partnerships between primary and community health and local authority services still remain. At the same time as developing relationships between them, both sets of partners have to effect major changes *within* their respective services. Primary care groups have to develop systems of clinical and organisational governance; local authorities are adopting corporate, rather than departmental, patterns of organisation and governance.[26] Local authorities will increasingly be expected to demonstrate 'best value' in purchasing and providing services, in which local communities and users will play a key consultative and regulatory role.[27] Primary and community health services, on the other hand, have relatively little experience of consulting and involving users.[28]

Problems of aligning boundaries and budgets for the people living within those boundaries, the continuing policy of charging for social, but not health, services, poorly developed information management and technology (IM&T) strategies and skills within both primary health and local authority services, and persistent prejudices and stereotypes derived from different organisational and professional cultures all present obstacles which remain to be overcome. Nevertheless, the renewed political commitment to partnership working is now underpinned by consistent performance management frameworks, greater budgetary and organisational flexibility and a modest injection of resources. This book is intended to contribute towards the translation of the vision of partnership into a reality.

REFERENCES

1   Department of Health (1997) *The New NHS: modern, dependable*, Cm 3807. The Stationery Office, London.

2   Department of Health (1998) *Partnership in Action: new opportunities for joint working between health and social services*. Department of Health, London.

3   Nocon A (1994) *Collaboration in Community Care in the 1990s*. Business Education Publishers, Sunderland.

4   Davies B, Bebbington A and Charnley H (1990) *Resources, Needs and Outcomes in Community Based Care: a comparative study of the production of welfare for elderly people in ten local authorities in England and Wales*. Avebury, Aldershot.

5   Department of Health (1995) *Joint Commissioning for Project Leaders*. HMSO, London.

6   NHSE (1994) *Developing NHS Purchasing and GP Fundholding*, EL(94)79. NHS Executive, Leeds.

7   Wistow G (1993) Aspirations and realities: community care at the crossroads. *Health and Social Care in the Community*. 3(4): 227–40.

8   Department of Health (1989) *Caring for People: community care in the next decade and beyond*, Cm 849. HMSO, London.

9   Craig G and Manthorpe J (1998) Small is beautiful? Local government reorganisation and the role of social services departments. *Policy and Politics*. 26(3): 189–207.

10 Gillam S (1994) *Community-oriented Primary Care*. King's Fund, London.

11 Dickson M, Wilkin D and Butler T (1998) *Practice-based Planning and Review: a case study of five sites*. National Primary Care Research and Development Centre, Manchester.

12 Myles S, Wyke S, Popay J, Scott J, Campbell A and Girling J (1998) *Total Purchasing and Community and Continuing Care: lessons for future policy development in the NHS*. King's Fund, London.

13 Bewley C and Glendinning C (1994) *Involving Disabled People in Community Care Planning.* Joseph Rowntree Foundation, York.

14 Department of Health (1998) *Our Healthier Nation: a contract for health,* Cm 3852. The Stationery Office, London.

15 Department of Health (1998) *Modernising Social Services: Promoting Independence, Improving Protection, Raising Standards,* Cm 4169. The Stationery Office, London.

16 NHSE (1997) *Health Action Zones – Invitation to Bid,* EL(97)65. NHS Executive, Leeds.

17 NCC (1995) *Charging Consumers for Services.* National Consumer Council, London.

18 Baldwin S and Lunt N (1996) *Charging Ahead: the development of local authority charging policies for community care.* Joseph Rowntree Foundation, York.

19 Hirst J (1998) Inequalities could outlive the wall. *Community Care.* 7 **May**: 6–7.

20 Cooper K (1998) Service mergers: who gains? *Community Care.* **9 April**: 10.

21 Le Mesurier N and Cumella N (1997) *The Lowesmoor Project.* Hereford and Worcester Social Services Department and Birmingham University.

22 Weir A (1999) Advice surgery. *Community Care.* **April**: 26–7.

23 ONS (1998*) Annual Abstract of Statistics, 1998 Edition.* Office of National Statistics, The Stationery Office, London.

24 Baldock J and Evers A (1992) Innovations in care for the elderly – the cutting edge of change for social welfare systems; examples from Sweden, the Netherlands and the United Kingdom. *Ageing and Society.* **12**(3): 289–312.

25 Department of Health (1997) *Better Services for Vulnerable People,* EL (97)62/CI(97)24. Department of Health, London.

26 Her Majesty's Government (1998) *Modern Local Government: in touch with the people,* Cm 4014. The Stationery Office, London.

27 DETR (1998) *Modernising Local Government: improving local services through best value.* Department of Environment, Transport and the Regions, London.

28 Audit Commission (1996) *What the Doctor Ordered: a study of GP fundholders in England and Wales.* The Stationery Office, London.

2

Strategic service partnerships: the experience of joint commissioning between primary health and social care

JOINT COMMISSIONING

As discussed in Chapter 1, the failure of health and local authorities to co-ordinate the planning and commissioning of health and social care services for older people is a long-standing problem. It results in gaps and overlaps in services, ineffective use of scarce resources and significant problems for patients, service users and their families. Since the mid-1990s, health and social services authorities have been encouraged to undertake joint commissioning,[1] to ensure the contracts which they negotiate with service providers are compatible and can thus help to integrate services at the level of individual users.[2]

There is no universally agreed definition of joint commissioning; the term can cover a wide range of activities. Department of Health (DoH) guidance suggests that commissioning is 'the strategic activity of assessing needs, resources and current services and developing a strategy as to how to best use available resources to meet need'. Joint commissioning is therefore 'the process in which two or more commissioning agencies act together to coordinate their commissioning, taking joint responsibility for translating strategy into action'.[1]

The key element which distinguishes joint commissioning from other partnership activities such as those described in Chapter 3 is that it has a *strategic* component involving assessment of needs, planning and the procurement of services to meet those needs. There must be some link between the commissioning activity and the development of services (although there is no prescribed process or pathway for this linkage).

To date, joint commissioning has tended to take place between health authorities and local authority social services departments, as the major health and social services budget holders respectively. However, this focus began to shift during the middle of the 1990s, with the explicit emphasis on a 'primary care-led NHS'.[3] GP fundholding, the extended budgets held by total purchasing pilot (TPP) projects and GP locality commissioning pilot projects all increased the profile of GPs and other primary care purchasers in purchasing and service commissioning. Indeed, some TPPs explicitly gave priority to the purchase and development of services at the health/ social care boundaries, although collaborative activities *with* local social services departments were slow to develop.[4]

The landscape of NHS purchasing and commissioning activities is currently undergoing further fundamental change, as responsibility for service commissioning is devolved to primary care groups (PCGs) and, increasingly from April 2000, to primary care trusts. The voluntary activities of fundholding and locality commissioning

GPs are, in effect, being extended across the whole of primary care. The requirement that all PCG boards include a representative from the local authority social services department is an important first step towards building strategic service planning and commissioning partnerships between primary and community health services and local authority social services. PCGs and trusts may eventually take over almost all the former commissioning responsibilities of health authorities, including responsibilities for joint commissioning of services with local authority partners. In the case of older people, the most significant of these partners are social services departments, although other statutory agencies (particularly local authority housing departments) may also come to play an increasingly important role in the commissioning of integrated community-based services for older people, and the voluntary and independent sectors will remain key providers of services.

The dominant role of health authorities in joint commissioning with local authorities during the earlier part of the 1990s means that there is still very little evidence of joint commissioning (either successful or unsuccessful) in which primary and community health services are involved as partners with local authority social services departments. This chapter presents evidence from some of the few 'leading edge' sites where primary and community health services have engaged in joint commissioning with local authority social services. This evidence base is very small, but nonetheless important. Indeed, instead of asking why primary health services have not been more involved in joint commissioning to date, it might be more appropriate to ask why it has happened at all.

- **Joint commissioning must involve strategic service development as well as operational collaboration between primary health and social care workers.**
- **Primary healthcare professionals and managers have not, to date, been widely involved in mainstream joint commissioning.**
- **Primary health services involvement in joint commissioning has so far been limited to a handful of projects.**

- **However, the role of primary and community health services in strategic service planning and commissioning partnerships is likely to increase through the development of PCGs and PCTs.**

The barriers to, and opportunities for, joint commissioning

There has been considerable research into the problems of joint planning and joint commissioning between health and social services authorities.[2,5] These barriers include a lack of common geographical boundaries, budgetary cycles and service development priorities, a failure to agree on shared, achievable goals at the outset of the process, mistrust derived from a lack of interprofessional understanding, and a lack of commitment and support from more senior managers in either or both organisations.[6] The introduction of markets into both NHS and local authority services also created additional barriers to collaboration, both between purchasers tempted to 'minimise market shares' (or 'cost-shunt') by passing funding responsibility on to other agencies, and between purchasers and provider organisations.[7]

Some of these problems may also inhibit the development of strategic partnerships between PCG/Ts and local authorities. For example, the populations served by PCGs are those registered with the GPs within each PCG; their distribution is unlikely to be coterminous with the geographic boundaries used by local authorities. Moreover, although most PCGs will be located within a single local authority, any social services department may have to relate to several PCGs. A further barrier arises from the competing pressures of internal organisational change and the development of relationships with other, external organisations. Local authorities will be required to implement major internal organisational changes over the next few years, while PCGs are likely to experience pressures to become Trusts. Both sets of internal changes will be demanding and will be subject to external scrutiny through audit and performance management; this may divert attention away from the development of partnerships and joint working.

On the other hand, a number of new measures may facilitate joint working. The development of health improvement plans (HImPs), to which the commitment of local authorities is also required, will provide a single, overarching framework within which both PCG/Ts and local authority services can develop common strategic objectives and service development priorities. The presence of a social services representative on each PCG board may prove a powerful factor in breaking down professional stereotypes and mistrust at the level of strategic service planning. The new statutory duty on all NHS organisations to work in partnership and the monitoring of partnership working by health authorities and NHSE regional offices is likely to secure the commitment of PCG/T members and senior managers alike. The new flexibilities described in Chapter 1, which were set out in *Partnership in Action*, are intended to support and extend closer relationships across the NHS–local authority boundary.

- **Barriers to joint working between health and social services have included different boundaries, different budgetary cycles and priorities, a lack of shared, achievable goals, interprofessional mistrust, and a lack of commitment from senior managers.**
- **Some of these barriers may continue to present problems for PCG/Ts. However, the commitment of local authorities to the local health improvement plan and social services representation on PCG boards may facilitate strategic joint working.**
- **The proposals contained in Partnership in Action will also extend and support NHS–local authority partnerships.**

Evidence to date from primary care involvement
in joint commissioning

The former total purchasing pilot projects (TPPs) gave GPs opportunities for purchasing all hospital and community health services for their patients, acting as a subcommittee of the local health authority. Of the 53 TPPs, 19 declared an interest in purchasing community or continuing healthcare services.[4] However, even these interested TPPs showed a marked lack of awareness of national community care policy: the GPs in the TPPs were more likely to be concerned about the co-ordination of services for individual patients and the service developments they initiated reflected this concern. Some TPPs negotiated access to a practice-based social worker or care manager, similar to the projects described in Chapter 3. Overall, within the lifetime of the pilots, TPPs demonstrated little success in commissioning integrated health and social care services for their populations. The TPPs tended to lack a population-based focus for their commissioning activities; moreover, service developments tended to reflect the interests of a lead GP and there was very little user or patient involvement in setting commissioning objectives.[4,8]

A series of GP locality commissioning pilot projects began in April 1998. Early evidence suggests that leaving strategic service development just to a few lead GPs is problematic.[9] Evaluation has already stressed the importance of involving *all* stakeholders in commissioning decisions, pointing out that this could be achieved through setting up subcommittees of the locality commissioning pilot projects. Both this and the TPP evaluation demonstrate the importance of securing sound internal structures and management before embarking on joint service commissioning with an outside agency. Both studies also highlight the relatively underdeveloped role of community nurses in commissioning services. Service development priorities tend to reflect those of GPs, even where supporting community nursing involvement was a declared intention.

The King's Fund has also worked closely with a small number of local projects to nurture the joint commissioning capacity of primary care.[10] This development work has highlighted the fragmented nature of primary health services – the networks of independent contractors and trusts, each with their own professional and managerial priorities. Consequently, joint commissioning has developed most easily where there has been enthusiasm from a number of articulate primary care professionals (usually GPs), some capacity for effecting service change (such as holding a budget) and a history of good joint working with local authority social services.[10]

The formation of primary care groups provides a potential framework for resolving the organisational fragmentation of primary and community healthcare. It seems clear from the limited evidence to date that this will be an essential basis for effective joint commissioning.

- **Primary care professionals, particularly GPs, are not necessarily aware of, or ready to tackle, national community care policies.**
- **GPs have had little experience to date of commissioning services to reflect population-based needs.**
- **The resolution of internal management issues for PCGs will be vital to the success of joint commissioning partnerships with outside agencies.**
- **The involvement of other primary care professionals, particularly community nurses, may be vital to the success of commissioning partnerships.**
- **The fragmented nature of primary care (which until now has been made up of disparate practices and trusts with no incentive to co-operate with each other) has been a significant barrier to joint commissioning.**

MODELS OF JOINT COMMISSIONING

Some of the initiatives referred to above do provide a valuable basis on which PCG/Ts can build. In particular, they allow us to identify three different models of joint commissioning:

- a quasi-single agency
- commissioning of specific services, and
- integrated primary health and social work teams.

In the *quasi-single agency* model, primary care professionals are involved with local authority purchasers in commissioning a wide range of health and social care (and sometimes other) services for all the patients living in a given area (for example, the area covered by a health authority or PCG). The model of *commissioning specific services* focuses on a narrower range of services, perhaps for a specific range of patients (such as frail older people). In the *integrated health and social care teams* model the focus is on the joint commissioning of health and social care services to improve access and co-ordination for individual users, rather than on strategic service development.

These three models reflect differences in the scope and range of joint commissioning activities: how far managers are involved as well as professionals; how far budgets are devolved and held by the key joint commissioning partners; how many services are being jointly commissioned; whether these are being commissioned for individuals, 'client' groups or whole populations; and whether the joint commissioning covers one or a cluster of services.

The three models therefore illustrate alternatives around which PCG/Ts and local authority social services departments might focus the development of their commissioning partnerships. Each model has its own particular advantages and shortcomings. The remainder of this chapter will describe these three different models, with illustrations from particular sites. With the end of GP fundholding and the development of PCGs, it is likely that some features of such 'trailblazing' projects will change. However, the aim here has been to identify the wider lessons which remain relevant to PCG/Ts.

A QUASI-SINGLE COMMISSIONING AGENCY

This model involves primary care professionals in the strategic planning and commissioning of services for the whole population within a given area. From April 2000, when the first *Partnership in*

Action sites go live, it will be possible for PCG/Ts and local authorities to pool their budgets or agree to one agency taking the lead in commissioning services. The experience of Easington (Table 2.1) demonstrates how primary care professionals, health and local authority staff can collaborate (along with other key local partners) in planning and commissioning a wide range of services for the whole community by acting as a *quasi-single commissioning agency*, even without these new flexibilities.

Lessons for primary care and health authority managers

Collaborative commissioning can entail some loss of power and autonomy for commissioning managers, whether at PCG/T or health authority level. An important source of compensation can be the clear benefits of collaboration for all parties involved.

Managers also need to be sufficiently committed to collaboration to devote the time and energy involved in building sustainable structures and relationships. Moreover, they need to extend this commitment to other potential stakeholders, in order to overcome historical tensions between primary health and social care agencies and professionals.

Some of the difficulties facing primary healthcare managers will already have been experienced by health authority managers in drawing up joint investment plans for continuing healthcare, rehabilitation and other services for vulnerable people, in conjunction with local authority partners. It will be important for the lessons and benefits of this experience to be communicated to primary care managers, to support them as they gradually take on responsibility for joint investment plans and other areas of joint commissioning.

However, some practical problems, such as those associated with the alignment of geographical boundaries, will continue to be experienced in primary care-level joint commissioning; solving these will require considerable skill and enthusiasm. The overarching objective of the Easington group was to create a specific focus on the needs of the *locality*, within which more co-ordinated health

Table 2.1: Easington Joint Commissioning Management Group

Description	• Locality-wide commissioning body responsible for commissioning all health and (with social services) social care services for 98 000 people living in Easington, County Durham, one of the most deprived areas in the North of England. • Formed to give a locality focus to commissioning in the area. This had previously been fragmented between three different health authorities, the county social services department and the local district council.
Funding	• Time contributed by service managers was funded by their respective organisations. • Time contributed by the Chair of the GP commissioning group was funded by the health authority. • A development officer post was initially funded by the King's Fund.
Management and structure	• Included representation from GP commissioning group, health authority, social services department, community health council, local advisory groups and district council. • Eight local advisory groups established by development officer, to maximise involvement of local people in planning and commissioning services.
Commissioning framework: services	• Main service developments arising from the commissioning group included pilot 'hospital at home' scheme, joint bathing service, stroke rehabilitation scheme and alignment of social workers/care managers with GP practices.
Key outcomes	• Successful focus on the needs of the Easington locality. • Improved interprofessional relationships between members of the group. • Reduction in historical tensions and boundary disputes between health and social care.

continued

Table 2.1: Continued

	• Improved provision of primary care in the locality through the shifting of services from secondary to primary care settings (e.g. provision of alarms for older people, and daycare services for elderly mentally ill patients).
Problems	• Early relationships among group members were tense as senior managers sought to protect their positions and influence over purchasing rather than collaborating in setting priorities.
	• Local advisory groups had problems in establishing roles and communication channels and involving stakeholders.
	• Some GPs felt disenfranchised by local advisory groups as they had no commissioning capacity.
	• GPs were represented by the Chair of GP commissioning group, but other primary care professionals weren't represented and didn't benefit from improved interagency and interprofessional working – a particular concern in relation to community nursing services.
Sustainability and transferability	• Initial funding and development support from the King's Fund.
	• Beyond the initial period, the support of key senior managers was essential in establishing the group as mainstream commissioning body.
	• Management and commissioning arrangements appeared well designed and adaptable.

Source: Smith J and Shapiro J (1996) *Evaluation of Easington Joint Commissioning Board: Some real wins for Easington.* Health Services Management Unit, University of Birmingham. Poxton R and Smith J (1997) Addressing health and social care in Easington: partnership in practice. *Community Care Planning and Review.* 5(5).

and social care services could be developed. In the Easington experience, this clear locality-focused objective created a common purpose and enabled the joint commissioning management group to become a mainstream strategic commissioning body. A similarly clear locality focus is also characteristic of PCG/Ts.

- **It takes time and energy to build up the relationships necessary for successful joint commissioning; responsibility for doing this will often fall on primary care and health authority managers. Commissioning managers often need to experience some benefits before they are willing to trust their counterparts and forego some of their power.**
- **Involving the right stakeholders is vital: they need to be sufficiently senior to be able to translate agreed priorities into service developments, and committed to the success of joint commissioning.**
- **The skill and enthusiasm of key managers is crucial to the success of joint commissioning, particularly in developing sustainable management and commissioning structures.**
- **The experiences of health authority managers in developing joint investment plans need to be shared with those involved in joint commissioning at primary care level.**
- **Budgets, priorities and responsibilities have to be agreed by all stakeholders early on in the commissioning process and attention paid to ways of overcoming differences between agencies in this area.**

Lessons for social services partners

To some extent, the lessons for social services commissioning partners mirror those of their health colleagues. Their sustained commitment will depend on the prospect of clear gains being achievable for all stakeholders. To some extent, the harmonisation of goals and objectives will be facilitated by local authorities' commitment to local health improvement plans; these can act as an overarching strategic framework for the commissioning activities of both social services and PCG/Ts.

However, local authority social services departments also have other statutory responsibilities – lead responsibilities in the assessment and provision of community care services under the 1990 NHS and Community Care Act and responsibilities for child protection and child welfare under the 1988 Children Act, for example. These responsibilities (which also often have a high public profile) are not shared by primary healthcare partners. Tensions may therefore arise between the statutory commitments of local authority social services partners and their commitments to partnerships with primary and community health services partners.

Although PCG/Ts will have increasing autonomy over their budgets (and considerably greater flexibility in the allocation of those budgets between different types of services), the budgetary flexibility of local authorities remains more constrained, partly by central government imposed spending limits and partly because of the statutory responsibilities referred to above. In addition, local authority partners are accountable to elected members for the allocation and spending of budgets, which may further restrict their flexibility in joint commissioning partnerships.

However, the participants in Easington were united in a common purpose of improving services in a deprived and hitherto underserved community. Without the development of this shared sense of purpose and common values it could have been far more difficult to sustain the involvement of key social services partners.

- **There need to be clear benefits for social services partners to legitimate and sustain their involvement in joint commissioning.**
- **Both the statutory responsibilities and local accountability of social services partners need to be acknowledged by their health colleagues.**
- **Shared goals and objectives are essential for sustaining the commitment of all partners.**

Lessons for primary care professionals

Some GPs in Easington felt alienated from the local advisory groups (which fed into the locality-wide management group), partly because they were not reimbursed for involvement in group activities and partly because (as non-fundholders) they had no resources to contribute to service developments. As one GP succinctly put it, 'there's no money in it'. For those GPs who retain independent contractor status, adequate reimbursement for activities like joint commissioning, which lie outside the provision of general medical services, will remain a key constraint. However, it may be easier to include involvement in joint commissioning partnerships as a contractual obligation for GPs employed on salaried contracts in personal medical services (PMS) pilot projects and as employees of PCTs.

On the positive side, evidence from Easington showed considerable gains for the GPs who were involved. They appreciated the opportunity to 'see the bigger picture' of the locality and its needs, rather than simply the needs of individual patients. They also valued the improved working relationships with both health and local authority managers, particularly when they also experienced tangible service developments as a result of this involvement (such as the alignment of care managers with GP practices).

The relative lack of involvement of other primary care professionals, particularly community nurses, was problematic in the Easington experience. This reflected the *provider* status assigned to community health services trusts within the NHS internal market. The requirement that PCGs include a community nursing representative on their boards, and the opportunities for integration of primary and community health services in primary care trusts are both likely to facilitate the involvement of these stakeholders in joint commissioning partnerships.

- **Appropriate contractual and/or financial support is essential for primary care professionals to take part in joint commissioning.**

- **Priority needs to be given to increasing the involvement and experience of nursing and other non-medical professionals in locality-based joint commissioning partnerships.**
- **Benefits to primary care professionals include a population-level perspective on health and social care needs, the opportunity to contribute to strategic service development, and improved interagency and inter-professional relationships.**

Lessons for patients and local communities

Encouraging local community involvement in service commissioning was one of the key aims of the Easington Joint Commissioning Group. Local advisory groups, covering smaller areas, were set up to facilitate this and the local community health council was also represented on the Joint Commissioning Group.

The local advisory groups had mixed success. There were problems establishing lines of communication and responsibilities, particularly as the groups had no budgets of their own. Local GPs also failed to engage with their local advisory groups and lay representatives on the Joint Commissioning Group reported feeling alienated from the main decision making.

- **Involving local people in locality-based joint commissioning partnerships requires specific objectives, commitment and some earmarked resources.**
- **In order to sustain local involvement, it must be perceived to be worthwhile. If there is no apparent link between lay involvement and strategic service development, then initial enthusiasm can quickly wane.**

A MODEL FOR JOINT COMMISSIONING OF SPECIFIC SERVICES

In this model primary care professionals collaborate with social services to commission a much narrower range of services for their patients. These are often key services considered to be at the boundaries between 'health' and 'social' care, such as bathing or personal care. In the example described in Table 2.2, the services were those identified by lead GPs as being problematic, namely the provision of care management and respite care for older patients. This model combined elements of both strategic service development (see above), with elements of an *integrated health and social care team* approach to commissioning for individual users (see below).

Lessons for primary care and health authority managers

As with broader, locality approaches to joint commissioning partnerships, securing agreement on geographical boundaries and definitions of eligible populations is essential. For example, a local authority social services department may allocate referrals of every-one over age 60 to its older people's services team, while primary care may wish to target services at over-75 year olds. Such differences in eligibility and access criteria – and their implications for the size of the budget contributed by respective partners – will need to be made explicit and compromises reached.

The experience of Bromsgrove shows that it is not always necessary for the health authority to act as enablers if primary care professionals can establish good working relationships on their own with social services colleagues. In Bromsgrove, the GPs in the TPP succeeded in joint commissioning with social services, despite the fact that relationships between the health and local authorities had historically been very poor. However, the converse is much

Table 2.2: Bromsgrove Total Purchasing Project

Description	• An early total purchasing pilot project which part-funded a team of care managers for older people based in the health centre and additional respite care facilities.
	• The TPP also part-funded a development manager to develop these jointly funded services.
Funding	• Resources were allocated to the TPP from the health authority on a capitation-based (rather than historical activity-based) formula.
	• Social services contributed part funding of care manager and development manager posts and respite care services from its mainstream budget; social services fully funded a manager for the care manager team.
Management and structure	• The joint-funded team of care managers for older people was managed by a social services-funded team manager.
	• A primary care manager (funded by the TPP) provided further management support for the project, maintaining the links between primary care professionals and care managers.
	• A development manager (jointly funded) was responsible for service development.
Commissioning framework: services	• Service developments included jointly funded respite care and multi-disciplinary seminars on stroke rehabilitation.
	• Practice-based care managers were able to improve access to home care services and residential services, but not commission any new service developments.
Key findings	• Interprofessional relationships between primary care professionals and social services workers were reported to be much improved.
	• Access to both health and social care services for older patients was speeded up by the team's ability to negotiate funding responsibilities quickly.

continued

Table 2.2: Continued

	• Primary care professionals could both contribute to strategic service developments and improve operational working relationships.
Problems	• GPs unable to influence the range or volume of mainstream social care services (especially home care).
	• Historic mistrust between health and social care workers had to be overcome by focused team-building.
	• Opportunities for collaborative commissioning on a broader range of mainstream health and social services remained underdeveloped.
Sustainability and transferability	• The patients registered with the cluster of GP practices in the TPP mainly fell within social services divisional boundaries and also approximated to the 'natural community' of Bromsgrove.
	• The size and level of management support within the TPP was directly comparable to those of many PCG/Ts.
	• There were social services concerns about the creation of inequities, because older people living in the TPP received an enhanced service compared with those in the rest of the local authority.

Source: Bosanquet N *et al.* (1998) *The Bromsgrove Total Purchasing Project 1994–1996.* Department of Primary Health and General Practice, Imperial College School of Medicine at St Mary's, London.

more likely – that a history of good joint working between the health and local authorities will form a sound basis on which joint commissioning can be devolved to PCG/T levels. It will, therefore, be important for health authority managers to share their experiences and support PCG/T members and managers in developing joint commissioning partnerships with social services.

- **Joint commissioning of specific services for older patients can be hindered by a lack of coterminous boundaries and different eligibility criteria.**
- **Where there is a history of trust and good joint working between health and social services authorities, health authority managers will need to share their expertise and support PCG/T members as partnership responsibilities are devolved.**

Lessons for social services

The Bromsgrove experience highlights a number of concerns. Social services partners may be anxious that NHS priorities (and the priorities of GPs in particular) will dominate the joint commissioning agenda. This concern may have been exacerbated by the total purchasing context of the Bromsgrove project, where the purchasing power of GPs was explicitly used to bring about service changes. The abolition of GP fundholding may therefore lessen this anxiety.

Initially, the Bromsgrove GPs did not appreciate the need for care managers based in their practices to work closely with a professional supervisor, so the social services department had to fund a team manager post to fulfil this role. The GPs also expected the care managers to be able to contribute to the strategic development of services, which they were unable to do because of their location at an operational, rather than strategic, level within their department. Social services, therefore, also part-funded a development manager to undertake strategic service development with primary care. A period of team building at the outset of the project was necessary to overcome some of these constraints.

The social services department covering Bromsgrove substantially realigned its pattern of service provision and the arrangements for older people to obtain community care assessments. This raised anxieties about a retreat from equity, as older people in the TPP were felt to be advantaged in obtaining social services compared to older people elsewhere in the local authority.

Despite the considerable financial and other contributions of the social services department, the success of the project was nevertheless 'owned' by GPs and the health authority, because it had arisen from a major experiment in primary care-led purchasing.

- **Where partnerships embrace both strategic and operational level matters, a period of team building is helpful in overcoming any misunderstandings of roles and responsibilities between primary care professionals and social services.**
- **Social services departments may be reluctant to engage in commissioning services which appear to privilege users in some parts of the authority compared with others.**
- **It is essential that both the failures and the successes of projects are 'owned' equally by both primary health and social services partners. The resource and other contributions of social services need to be fully acknowledged.**

Lessons for primary health professionals

Because the Bromsgrove project was intrinsically linked to an early total purchasing pilot project, the priorities and concerns of GPs (for example, to obtain swifter access to community and respite care services in order to reduce length of hospital stay) tended to dominate the service development agenda. However, as the experiences of other total purchasing pilot projects and the locality commissioning pilot projects also show, it cannot be assumed that these concerns necessarily reflect the views of all local GPs nor the needs of local people; the priorities articulated by 'lead' GPs need to be discussed more widely.

The Bromsgrove experience also illustrates the value of involving social services colleagues as partners right from the start. The GPs expressed some frustration at not being able to develop social services-funded home care services in the ways they would have liked, but this may have obscured opportunities for other service developments which could have been achieved through closer joint working.

In Bromsgrove, as in many other TPPs, there was no significant involvement of non-GP primary care professionals, particularly community nurses, in the commissioning of services. This is a major shortcoming which will need to be overcome, particularly if this model is to be transferable to primary care trusts, in which community health services may be expected to play a substantial role in strategic planning and commissioning.

- **Primary care professionals, particularly GPs, need to ensure that service commissioning involves all relevant stakeholders and reflects local needs.**
- **It is important to secure the commitment of social services to enable 'joint' commissioning to take place. This could significantly improve the capacity to affect service provision in areas affecting the work of primary care, such as the provision of intensive home care.**
- **Particular attention needs to be paid to supporting the role of community nurses in commissioning specific services.**

The lack of patient involvement

Older patients at Bromsgrove benefited from access to the additional health and social care services commissioned by the project, such as GP beds to enable earlier hospital discharge and the jointly funded respite care service. They also enjoyed faster access to community care assessments and services, because of the improved communication and interprofessional relations between primary care professionals (notably GPs) and care managers in the project.

However, patients did not have any significant involvement in planning these developments. Primary care services have a poor tradition of involving patients in service development priorities and, unlike the other initiatives described in this chapter, Bromsgrove had no dedicated development input to increase lay or user stakeholder involvement.

Although new services were developed, there was also no evidence that existing health and social care services were better co-ordinated for individual users. Primary care professionals also reported that the levying of charges for social services restricted the development of 'seamless' packages of services.

- **Patients in this model can benefit from enhanced access to a wider range of health and social care services.**
- **However, the lack of patient involvement in service development calls into question how far these new services reflect patients' own priorities.**

INTEGRATED HEALTH AND SOCIAL CARE TEAMS

One of the problems faced by older people and their families is a lack of co-ordination between health and social care services. For example, older people receiving both nursing and home care may find information is not passed between the two services, or that assessment and review processes are duplicated. Some of these problems can be overcome if primary health and social care services are provided by joint or integrated teams of community nursing staff, care managers, home care workers and therapists, who are based in the GP practice or health centre (Table 2.3).

There is an important distinction between this model and the GP practice-attached social workers described in Chapter 4. In the integrated health and social care teams described here, the *commissioning* of services for individual patients is integrated, through a single assessment and care management process; thus primary health professionals can assess for and commission social services

Table 2.3: Malmesbury Integrated Community Care Team

Description	• An integrated primary health and social care team based in a GP practice in Malmesbury, Wiltshire. • Social workers, occupational therapists and community nurses all carried out community care assessments; service packages were approved by a team manager, employed by social services.
Funding	• Professionals were funded by their respective organisations. • Initial development of the team was supported by King's Fund.
Management and structure	• A steering group managed the project with input from the GP practice, health authority and social services. • Team leader was a social services manager with power to approve spending on services for individuals.
Commissioning framework: services	• Primary care professionals who had undergone training could act as care managers, assess and obtain both health and social care services for their patients. • No opportunities for strategic service commissioning.
Key findings	• Improved access to services for patients. • Improved interprofessional understanding and communication. • Fewer delays in getting assessments and services because of improved communication. • Primary care professionals gained additional skills and expertise.
Problems	• Initial team building necessary to overcome interprofessional barriers. • Difficult to sustain user and carer involvement beyond the project's initial stage. • No measurable differences in service outcomes for users or carers.

continued

Table 2.3: Continued

Sustainability and transferability	• Health authority, primary healthcare and social services have history of good relations and innovative joint working in Wiltshire. Replicating this project would be more difficult where relationships are less good. • Other methods of improving frontline operational partnerships (e.g. employing link workers, attaching care managers to GP practices) have been shown to deliver similar improvements in access to services and communication.

Source: Tucker C and Brown L (1997) *Evaluating Different Models for Jointly Commissioning Community Care.* Report No 4. The Wiltshire Social Services and University of Bath Research and Development Partnership, Bath.

and vice versa. This is why it is described here as a model of joint commissioning.

Lessons for health managers

A history of good working relations between health authority, primary care and social services managers was considered vital to the success of this project. The health authority had already supported a number of other innovations (e.g. the joint-funded appointment of 'link workers') to improve communications between primary care professionals and social services.

Integrated teams require agreement on the geographical boundaries served by the project. This may be easier to achieve in smaller communities or rural areas than in metropolitan areas, where a GP's patients can be scattered across a number of social services divisional offices or even between different local authorities.

This model of joint commissioning requires good project management, including networking and facilitation skills. Because of the localised nature of integrated teams, project managers may also need to devote attention to 'advertising' the benefits of an integrated team, so that the model can be 'rolled out' across a wider locality.

- **A history of good working relationships between health authorities, social services and primary care is important to the success of this model.**
- **Good project management is needed and work may be needed to 'roll out' successful projects to neighbouring primary health settings.**

Lessons for social services

If integrated health and social care teams are based in primary care, social services staff may fear that their work will be dominated by the concerns of primary and community health staff. However, this was avoided in Malmesbury by investing in an initial programme of sustained team building, supported by the King's Fund. The project was therefore jointly 'owned' by both primary care professionals and social services.

Although social services bore some additional costs of the team (such as the extra travelling undertaken by the team manager between the GP practice and social services office), they also benefited from the fact that primary care professionals could carry out community care assessments, a task previously only performed by social services staff.

The integrated teams also reduced or removed delays in obtaining the contributions of community nurses and therapists to community care assessments; social workers did not need to request and then wait for the input of health professionals to multidisciplinary assessments. Delays in obtaining primary and community health service contributions to complex 'packages' of care (for example, home care and nursing services to support a patient's discharge from hospital) also helped the work of social services.

- **An initial period of team building can ensure that both social services and primary healthcare professionals feel they 'own' the project.**

- **Social services can benefit from having additional trained care managers able to carry out community care assessments.**
- **Social services staff found it easier to obtain community nursing contributions to multi-disciplinary assessments and nursing and therapy services for older people.**

Lessons for primary care teams

Integrated health and social care teams can significantly enhance both the size and the effectiveness of the primary healthcare team; the team gains both additional members and quicker access to a range of social care services.

Community nurses and therapists are integral members of joint health and social care teams – far more so than in the other two models of joint commissioning described above. The opportunities for community nurses and frontline social care staff to work closely together were considered particularly valuable in Malmesbury. Other members of the primary healthcare team, such as practice nurses, also reported benefits from the closer collaboration with community nursing.

The community nurses who were members of the integrated team reported increased job satisfaction from their enhanced role. Although initial difficulties were experienced because of the different working methods of nurses and social workers, these were gradually overcome through the shared commitment to successful joint working.

- **The integrated team gave community nurses a key role in commissioning services for individual patients.**
- **Community nurses reported increased job satisfaction as a result of their enhanced role in carrying out community care assessments.**
- **The primary healthcare team was extended and delays in accessing both health and social care services were reduced.**

Lessons for patients

Service users were involved in the planning and establishment of the Malmesbury integrated team, as part of the King's Fund's preliminary development work. Some patients expressed concern that moving social services into a primary healthcare setting would result in services becoming 'medicalised' in their outlook and approach. Disabled service users were particularly concerned about this risk and the possible threat to their rights to services to support independent living. Users also expressed anxiety that a single integrated team would reduce their choice of services and entry points to those services.

However, the benefits to patients appeared to outweigh these concerns. Access to services was speeded up, duplicate assessments were eliminated and the length of time taken to put services in place was reduced, because of the improved communication between health and social care professionals.

It was, nevertheless, difficult to sustain the involvement of service users beyond the initial development phase of the project. Healthcare professionals in particular were resistant to users being involved in routine operational meetings because of threats to patient confidentiality, and it was difficult to find acceptable alternative ways of involving users in the working of the team.

- **Patients were concerned about the possible medicalisation of social care services.**
- **Patients experienced easier and quicker access to community care assessments and services and improved co-ordination of multiple service 'packages'.**
- **Development support at the start of the project enabled users and carers to be involved in setting the team's aims and object-ives, but it was difficult to sustain this involvement.**

PRIMARY CARE GROUPS AND TRUSTS: THE POTENTIAL FOR JOINT COMMISSIONING WITH SOCIAL SERVICES PARTNERS

All three of the joint commissioning models described above provide valuable models for primary care groups and trusts. The models differ in terms of the range of services which are jointly commissioned and the size and composition of the populations for whom they were being commissioned. These are the kinds of parameters on which decisions will need to be taken in setting up any joint commissioning partnership between PCG/Ts and local authority social services departments. Exactly where the parameters are set will probably depend on the PCG/T's 'level' and upon the previous history of partnership working with the local authority.

The only aspect of the three models described above which is likely to be less relevant to PCG/Ts is where, for example in the Malmesbury integrated health and social care team, commissioning partnerships operate solely at the level of the individual GP practice. Even though the joint commissioning of specific services in Bromsgrove was based upon a GP total purchasing pilot project, in practice the number of GPs involved in the pilot and the population which it covered approximated to a smaller PCG. It is unlikely, however, that either PCGs or their social services partners will wish to promote isolated practice-level commissioning partnerships, unless these are accompanied by a clear commitment to 'rolling out' in the longer term.

The new PCG/T context will enable some of the problems identified in the three models above to be resolved. For example, some of the GPs in the Easington area felt disenfranchised from the locality commissioning group because they did not have the 'leverage' of a budget; conversely the significant service developments in Bromsgrove could be in part ascribed to the budgetary autonomy and flexibility of its TPP status. All

PCGs of course have budgets over which they will be able to exercise increasing control; this should help to equalise and enhance primary care relationships with local authority social services partners.

Commissioning partnerships will also be assisted by the statutory duty placed on PCG/Ts to work in partnership with local authority and other service providers, and by the gradual inclusion of indicators of partnership working into the routine performance management of PCG/Ts. However, it will take time for PCGs to acquire skills and expertise effectively to execute these new responsibilities, given primary care's relative lack of involvement in joint commissioning to date. In the meantime, it will be vitally important for health authority managers experienced in joint commissioning (especially in developing joint investment plans) to provide support to PCGs, so that their expertise and experience can be devolved along with their budgets.

The three models of partnership commissioning involve the various groups of primary care professionals to very different degrees. Given the emphasis on GP-led purchasing and commissioning during the early part of the 1990s, it is perhaps not surprising that two of the three models were centred on decision making between GPs and social services partners; community nursing staff played little or no role in commissioning. This balance is one which will need to change, particularly as PCGs move towards full Trust status. The advantages of involving community nurses in commissioning activities, particularly the improvement in service co-ordination, can be clearly seen in the Malmesbury example (Table 2.3).

The involvement of patients, service users, local communities and carers in the examples of joint commissioning described above was very patchy. Primary care traditionally has relatively little experience in this area; significantly, the involvement of users and carers in setting objectives for the Malmesbury integrated health and social care team was facilitated by the King's Fund. However, this is an area in which PCGs have much to learn from their local authority partners, who since 1992 have been fulfilling a statutory duty to consult users and carers in the preparation of their plans for community care services.

Finally, it is important to stress that all three of the models described above were developed without the flexibility offered by pooled budgets. All three (even the integrated health and social care team) also managed to negotiate the thorny problem of how to assess and collect charges for social care, but not NHS, services. These issues are often cited as examples of major barriers to joint working. The initiatives described here all managed to overcome these problems. The overarching 'lesson' is that commissioning partnerships can succeed through hard work and commitment, rather than being dependent on sweeping legislative changes. Indeed, it is arguable that the development of joint commissioning partnerships is an essential foundation on which the *Partnership in Action* flexibilities can effectively be built.

REFERENCES

1 Department of Health (1995) *An Introduction to Joint Commissioning.* Department of Health, London.

2 Poxton R (1996) Bridging the gap: joint commissioning of health and social care. In: Hamson A (ed) *Healthcare UK (1995/6)*. King's Fund, London.

3 NHSE (1994) *Developing NHS Purchasing and GP Fundholding,* EL(94)679. NHS Executive, Leeds.

4 Myles S, Wyke S, Popay J, Scott J, Campbell A and Girling J (1998) *Total Purchasing and Community and Continuing Care: lessons for future policy development in the NHS*. King's Fund, London.

5 Nocon A (1994) *Collaboration in Community Care in the 1990s.* Business Education Publishers, Sunderland.

6 Hardy B, Turrell A and Wistow G (1992) *Innovations in Community Care Management*. Avebury, Aldershot.

7 House of Commons Health Committee (1998) *The Relationship Between Health and Social Services: first report.* The Stationery Office, London.

8 Mays N, Goodwin N, Killoran A and Malbon G (1998) *Total Purchasing: a step towards primary care groups.* King's Fund, London.

9 Regen E, Smith J and Shapiro J (1998) *First off the Starting Block: lessons from GP commissioning pilots for primary care groups.* Health Services Management Centre, University of Birmingham, Birmingham.

10 Poxton R (1999) *Partnerships in Primary and Social Care: integrating services for vulnerable people.* King's Fund, London.

3

Frontline collaboration between primary care and social services workers

The previous chapter discussed the experiences of strategic collaboration between primary care professionals and social services in the planning and commissioning of services for older people. It identified some of the barriers and challenges which will face PCG/Ts as they embark on collaborative commissioning of services with their partners in local authorities.

However, as was pointed out in that chapter, those models of joint commissioning which offer the most gains in developing new strategic patterns of services are less likely to be able to tackle the day-to-day problems created by poor collaboration between front-line professionals working with older people in the community. While health and social services managers may succeed in securing joint funding for, say, a new respite care service, this will not benefit the hard-worked GP who is unable to obtain routine feedback on the referrals he or she makes to social services, or the busy social services care manager who is unable to make contact with district nurses to carry out joint assessments. Above all, it is at the frontline of service delivery where patients in the community most often suffer from a lack of co-ordination between health and social services professionals. For example, frail older people and others with a range of complex needs may experience duplicate assessments by different professionals, or problems in obtaining comprehensive information about services, if there is poor communication between the different health and social services professionals about their respective responsibilities and activities.

Close collaboration at this level is therefore important for older people and primary health and social care profesionals. This chapter will discuss how to improve frontline collaboration between primary health and social care professionals. It will focus particularly on the most common strategy for improving frontline collaboration: designating a social services worker to liaise with primary care professionals and/or basing a social worker in the primary care team (usually a GP surgery) on a sessional or full-time basis.

COMMUNITY CARE FOR OLDER PEOPLE

It is important throughout this chapter to bear in mind the changing roles of local authority social services staff, particularly where services for frail older people are concerned. With the implementation of major community care changes in 1993, considerable importance was attached to the development of 'care management'. Social services staff in effect act as micro-commissioners, assessing needs and constructing 'packages' of appropriate services from a number of potential sources, rather than simply allocating a standard service package regardless of older people's aspirations and choices. This is partly intended to ensure that service users received more individualised services which are tailored to meet their needs and circumstances. It is also intended to facilitate a greater involvement of independent sector organisations in providing services and thereby extending the range of private, voluntary and in-house services available to older people and their families.[1]

However, because of growing financial constraints on local authority budgets, assessment has increasingly been used as a mechanism for prioritising needs and restricting access to services for all but those deemed most at risk.[2] Indeed, many social services departments now ration access to assessment itself, through a range of managerial and bureaucratic procedures which effectively delay or circumvent the assessment and care management process for all but those considered to be at the greatest risk of harm.[3]

In relation to frail older people, therefore, the role of social services staff has changed considerably. The main activities of care managers are now focused on assessing needs and making referrals or recommendations for services such as meals on wheels, home care, day care and short- or long-term residential or nursing home care. These services are frequently purchased from a range of different in-house and independent organisations. This can create additional problems if the actual provision of home care or respite care services is contracted out to private or voluntary sector organisations. Primary care professionals, particularly community nurses, may consequently need to liaise with multiple social care providers over the provision of services and the monitoring of older people in poor health.

Moreover, with continuing pressures on local authority budgets, the allocation of these services is likely to be governed by authority-wide guidelines on urgency, levels of risk and maximum cost ceilings for any individual client. In addition, applicants for services are also likely to have to undergo a financial assessment and pay charges for any social care services that they receive. The Audit Commission has found considerable variation between local authorities in the following areas: the proportion of older people referred for community care services who receive a full assessment; the maximum amount of money that local authorities are willing to spend on domiciliary services for individual older people; and the average level of home care and home help-type services provided to individual households.[4] This variation further emphasises the importance of close collaboration at local levels. Primary care professionals need to have accurate information about their *own* local authority's priorities and policies to be able to make appro-priate referrals and give their patients the right information.

ADDRESSING THE HEALTH/SOCIAL CARE DIVIDE: OVERCOMING ORGANISATIONAL AND PROFESSIONAL BARRIERS TO COLLABORATION

There are both benefits and pitfalls associated with setting up and running collaborative ventures involving frontline staff. Making the potential costs and gains clear enables us to judge whether a new initiative is a 'success' (i.e. it managed to overcome or alleviate some or all of the barriers) or a 'failure' (i.e. it did not). Further details of how to evaluate new collaborative initiatives can be found in Chapter 4.

Most discussions of barriers to collaboration tend to treat organisational, professional and interpersonal barriers separately.[5,6] While this may be useful from the perspective of policy analysis, it may be less helpful from the perspectives of individual professionals, who are likely to experience several of these problems at once. For example, a common complaint from primary care professionals is the difficulty they experience in obtaining information and feedback following a referral to social services. This could be due to organisational barriers (such as the length of time which older people at low risk must wait before receiving a full assessment), professional barriers (such as a social worker's concern to maintain client confidentiality), or interpersonal barriers (for example, mutual differences in attitudes and perceptions between individual social services and primary care staff). This chapter has therefore approached the issue of frontline collaboration from the perspectives of the different professionals involved, rather than following conventional analytic distinctions.

Barriers to frontline collaboration from the perspectives of managers in primary health and local authority services

From this perspective, it is most often the failure to adequately plan collaborative ventures, ensuring that all the stakeholders are involved and committed to the project, which acts as a barrier to collaboration. Planning needs to take into account the fact that local authorities and NHS organisations have different funding streams, budgetary cycles, management structures and accountability arrangements; these can impose very considerable barriers to joint working at all levels and do not lend themselves easily to marginal transfers of responsibility and funding in the light of local agreements and arrangements.[7] *The New NHS: modern, dependable* did not address these major barriers, and although some of the *Partnership in Action* flexibilities may help alleviate them, it will only do so in those areas which use them, and will not address all the barriers.

For example, because local authority services are funded in part through local taxation, the managers of these services are accountable to locally elected members, who may also play a major role in determining overall spending priorities. The new 'best value' regime in local authorities also seeks to increase democratic accountability, both in relation to the setting of overall service priorities and in ensuring the delivery of high quality services.[8] The new local government White Paper proposes the extension of these principles across local government services as a whole.[9]

In contrast, NHS managers have very weak accountability obligations, certainly so far as democratic accountability is concerned. Indeed, it has been argued that developments in NHS policies over the past decade have strengthened the emphasis on NHS managers reporting upwards to the NHS Executive and the Secretary of State for Health, rather than outwards to local communities.[10] Some of the differences between NHS and local authority accountability structures may slowly diminish, with the prospect of both local authorities and health authorities eventually being subject to common strategic objectives as set out in local health improvement plans[11] and National Priorities Guidance.[12] However, neither the development of common strategic objectives nor the imposition of common performance frameworks across the health/social services interface[12] is likely to narrow the gap between the two service sectors with respect to their different traditions of accountability to local communities.

Consequently, local authority managers may be viewed by their health colleagues as having insufficient flexibility or budgeting autonomy, particularly in relation to small-scale, practice-level initiatives. Even the larger populations to be served by PCG/Ts may be considerably smaller than those of the local authority area as a whole; again, social services managers will be accountable to elected members for the equitable distribution of resources and services across this wider population.

A further problem for managers is the lack of common geographical boundaries between GP practices, PCG/Ts and local authorities (or local authority divisions). *The New NHS: modern, dependable* requires PCG/Ts to take account of local authority as well as health authority boundaries.[11] However, there is little evidence that this imperative is shaping the development of PCG/Ts, and the situation is further complicated by the fact that GP practice lists are only loosely geographically based and contain an element of self-selection of patients within an area. It may therefore be very difficult for local authority managers to determine which particular service divisions or local offices should most appropriately liaise with any one GP practice. Indeed, this will be a particular problem in urban areas, where any social services divisional office may need to liaise with half a dozen or more GP practices and their teams, or where a particular practice draws its patients from across two or more local authority boundaries.

Finally, there are likely to be differences in the expenditure priorities for health and local authority services. For example, because of their statutory duties under the 1989 Children Act and the pressures emanating from the joint Audit Commission/Social Services Inspectorate joint reviews of social services, a major priority for many local authorities is to improve their services for children and families considered to be at risk. In contrast, continuing political pressures to reduce hospital waiting lists mean that for primary care partners, a major priority will be ensuring that frail older people have speedy access to those services which can prevent hospital admission or support early discharge.

As mentioned above, these differences may become less marked over time, as local authorities align their strategic priorities with those of the local health improvement programme. However, they look set to continue for the immediate future. It is significant that the priorities for interagency working which have been set for local authority social services departments up to 2001/2 are focused on young offenders, crime reduction and sure start programmes,[12] none of which is likely to be a priority for NHS partners.

None of these barriers are insurmountable. As this chapter will show, provided that certain key 'success factors' are followed, it should certainly be possible to plan and implement closer collaboration at the front line between primary health and social care services. Most collaborative projects which fail do so because of poor planning and a lack of shared ownership at the outset. These pitfalls can only be avoided if the barriers to collaboration are acknowledged and addressed at an early stage.

- **Primary health and social services partners need to acknowledge and respect the different accountability structures of the NHS and local authorities.**
- **The difficulties caused by a lack of common boundaries need to be overcome and efforts need to be made to achieve greater co-terminosity.**
- **The differing priorities and budgeting cyles of health and local authority managers need to be recognised.**

Barriers to frontline collaboration for primary care professionals

One of the biggest barriers to collaboration between frontline primary health and social services professionals within a primary care setting may be a lack of collaboration between primary healthcare professionals themselves. Whilst reference is often made to the 'primary healthcare team', many commentators argue that this is misleading, in view of the lack of cohesion which can exist between the different professionals who constitute the 'team'.[13] This can be attributed to a variety of factors, but one of the most important may be the differences in financial, contractual and professional status between GPs and other members of the team.

GPs have stoutly defended their status as independent contractors, remunerated according to a complicated national formula, since the creation of the NHS.[14] Associated with this tradition is the 'small business'[15] culture of general practice. This, and the emphasis within the profession on the quality of the GP–patient relationship, has tended to create a dominant culture of individualism, which may fail to recognise the organisational and managerial frameworks within which other primary care professionals are employed. It is only recently that a salaried option has been introduced in a limited number of Primary Care Act pilot site projects.[16] It is possible that the collaboration *between* GPs, which is required by their common membership of PCG/Ts, will also modify this individualism in the longer term. However, *The New NHS: modern, dependable* reiterated that the independent contractor status would remain unaltered for the majority of GPs.

On the other hand, nursing and other primary care professionals all have employee status, albeit with different employers and therefore managers. Practice nurses and clerical staff are employed by GP practices; other professionals such as counsellors may also be employed by the practice on a sessional basis. In contrast, community health staff tend to be employed by Trusts. *The New NHS: modern, dependable* envisages the eventual formation of *Primary Care Trusts* to replace the old GP practice/NHS trust divide and this may offer an organisational route to breaking down the barriers to collaboration between GPs, other primary health-care professionals and community nurses. The uptake of the salaried GP option under Primary Care Act pilot sites is also set to continue and will further reduce professional differences within the primary care team. However, it will be some time before it is clear whether this will also lead to the development of more cohesive primary healthcare teams.

A lack of collaboration between primary care professionals can exacerbate difficulties in collaborating with social services staff. The success of some frontline collaboration projects has been limited because the social services staff have been unable to forge effective links with one or more key primary care professionals. This could be a GP who is less committed to the project than her/his partners, a community nursing team which is marginalised in the initial planning of the project, or a practice manager who is not involved in discussing how the project might affect his/her work.

Even where relations within the extended primary healthcare team are good, other barriers to collaboration between primary health and social services staff may still cause problems. Often these simply arise from a mutual lack of understanding of each other's professional ethos and responsibilities. Primary health professionals may be perceived by social services staff as bound by medical models of assessing needs, deciding on appropriate service interventions and delivering those services, which are not aligned with social objectives of enhancing independence and safety or combating social exclusion. In contrast, social services staff may be perceived as being too slow in responding to referrals, or as following rigid bureaucratic rules in the allocation of services.

One of the criteria for measuring the success of a collaborative project must therefore be how far it can overcome mutual mistrust and improve understanding of the professional and organisational differences between the primary healthcare team and social services staff.

- **Collaborative ventures have a greater chance of success if they are built upon a history of successful team working between primary healthcare professionals.**
- **Problems in collaboration can be caused by GPs' independent contractor status; it may be easier to bring GPs into closer collaboration with frontline social services staff using the new salaried employment options for GPs.**
- **Differences between 'social' and 'medical' approaches to working with patients need to be recognised and respected.**
- **Mistrust and misunderstandings between health and social services staff need to be addressed and overcome through investment in information-sharing and team-building exercises.**

Barriers to frontline collaboration for social services staff

Of course, many of the barriers experienced by primary care professionals apply equally to social services staff attempting to work more closely with them. However, for social services staff, collaboration may be impeded by some additional professional and organisational barriers.

Unlike doctors, nurses and other healthcare workers, social workers do not yet have an independent professional body which provides a code of conduct to regulate their day-to-day practice and training. The 1998 White Paper *Modernising Social Services* recommended the establishment of a General Social Services Council, which would eventually be able to provide the same kind of professional regulation for social workers and other social care staff as currently exists for doctors and nurses. In the meantime, social workers' professional standards are maintained through line management supervision arrangements. It is, therefore, not currently possible for social workers to become entirely independent of their professional colleagues, even though they are based in primary care premises and work closely with primary care professionals.

The need for social workers to maintain close contact with their professional colleagues and employing organisations has been increased by the duties placed on local authorities by the 1990 NHS and Community Care Act. This gave social services departments statutory responsibility for assessing needs and allowing access to local authority-funded residential, domiciliary and day care services. Tight constraints on local authority spending since the implementation of the Act have meant that access to both needs assessments and subsequent service provision tend to be restricted to those with the most urgent needs. Individual social services workers are therefore obliged to operate within criteria of eligibility for assessments and services, and also within their authorities' capped budgets for community care services. Budgets are sometimes devolved to local area team levels; in other cases they are the responsibility of individual care managers. There is usually a ceiling on the amount which can be spent on any individual client – beyond that, a special case may have to be made to the local authority social services committee. Social services workers, therefore, may appear to be unduly constrained by bureaucratic procedures, simply because they must work within their local authority's eligibility criteria and budget constraints. The development of devolved, cash-limited budgets for PCG/Ts may in the long term reduce this gulf in the levels of autonomy of primary care and social services professionals to obtain services for individual older people, as primary care professionals are also likely to find themselves working within PCG-set cash limits.

- **Adequate arrangements for the professional supervision of practice (or community health team) based social services workers need to be in place in order to avoid professional isolation and losing touch with changing departmental policies and procedures.**

Barriers to frontline collaboration for individual patients

Although patients often benefit from successful collaborative projects, one of the biggest barriers to success from their point of view is that the projects themselves do not reflect a significant degree of user or patient consultation. Involving patients from the outset in the planning and running of collaborative projects is rare, perhaps reflecting a lack of experience on the part of primary care professionals in involving and consulting patients in the organisation and delivery of health services. Social services departments have a longer, and sometimes more successful, history in involving service users in service innovations (although many user organisations would claim that there is still some progress to be made).[17] However, this expertise may not be brought into play if collaborative projects are initiated by primary care professionals or the health authority, rather than from social services departments.

A lack of patient involvement at the outset of projects can mean that managers and practitioners are unaware of patients' needs and priorities. They may consequently set projects up which reflect either their own professional and organisational needs, or their *perceptions* of what patients need (which may not tally with patients' own perceptions of their needs).

- **Collaborative ventures are more likely to meet the needs of patients and their families if the latter are properly consulted on the design and involved in the management of the project.**
- **Primary care professionals may have less experience than their social care colleagues in consulting and involving patients in the planning and delivery of services.**

Co-location/attachment schemes within a primary care setting

As was discussed above, there are many different types of collaborative projects involving health and social care workers located in primary care settings. The most common is the co-location, attachment or alignment of social care workers with a GP practice, and it is this example that will be used to highlight the means of creating successful frontline collaboration.

Many examples of these types of schemes have been piloted since the implementation of the 1990 NHS and Community Care Act, and some of them have been well documented. In this section, four case studies will be briefly described (Tables 3.1–3.4), and the lessons from them and other similar schemes will be discussed.

Table 3.1: Practice-based care management in Greenwich

Description	• Three care managers, employed by Greenwich Social Services, based in a GP practice (two of the care managers covered more than one practice).
Funding	• Through the London Implementation Zone Initiative.
Management of project	• Developmental project steering group, meeting monthly, with health authority, social services, voluntary sector, community health council and evaluators/trainers represented.
Supervision and management of care managers	• Each post had a 'project team', consisting of the project manager, practice-based care manager, support worker, GP and social services manager, who carried out operational management.
	• Professional supervision provided by line manager in social services department (SSD) district office.
Day-to-day running	• Referrals for all practice patients were received by the care managers from health workers at the practice, social services department, patients and their families.
	• Care managers used SSD eligibility criteria and budgets when accessing services for patients, but had flexibility in prioritising their workloads.

continued

Table 3.1: Continued

Key findings	• Improved communication and professional co-operation. • Greater job satisfaction for care managers. • Better holistic and joint assessments of patients' needs. • Improved response time and throughput of cases. • Increased patient satisfaction – viewed as improvement over 'bureaucracy' of standard SSD.
Problems	• Project viewed as part of the NHS by primary care professionals, failing to acknowledge contribution of SSD. • There was insufficient back-up when care managers were on sick/annual leave. • Varying commitment from primary care professionals meant that the care managers often had to work long hours to ensure that everyone was involved and informed.
Sustainability and transferability	• In its pilot form the project proved too expensive for the SSD to sustain or extend. • An alternative model of 'aligning' care managers to practices is planned. • Further developments are to be planned 'incrementally'.

Source: Hodgson C R (1997) *It's All Good Practice: evaluating practice-based care management in Greenwich.* South East Institute of Public Health.

Table 3.2: Social workers attached to GP practices in Derby

Description	• 1.5 full-time equivalent (FTE) social workers attached to five inner city GP practices in Derby, to work with the elderly, disabled and mentally ill.
Funding	• Through joint finance.
Management of project	• No steering group.
Supervision and management of care managers	• Social workers received supervision from line managers in district team, but were 'divorced' from the team.

continued

Table 3.2: Continued

Day-to-day running	• One full-time social worker covered three GP practices, one part-time social worker covered two GP practices. • Referrals received from primary care professionals, patients and their families. • After the workload became unmanageable, it was agreed that the district team would take some referrals; however, this did not work in practice and the social workers had to manage their increased workload. • Initially the hours of the half-time social worker were set by the SSD; however, this did not fit with surgery hours so they were changed to be more convenient for GPs. • Work was not mainly care management, but counselling or benefits advice, which was not seen as the 'core' work of a social worker. Care management was usually undertaken by a worker in the district team rather than the practice-attached social worker.
Key findings	• Primary care professionals perceived a reduction in paperwork, quicker response times and easier access to social workers. • Improved working relationships between primary care professionals and social workers, particularly between district nurses and social workers. • Easier and quicker referrals for patients and reduced stigma (because the social worker was viewed as being part of the primary care team). • Job satisfaction for social workers due to autonomy over day-to-day work. • Primary care professionals felt there was better feedback from referrals.
Problems	• Insufficient preparation at outset meant there were no clear guidelines for the social worker's role, and many members of the primary healthcare team (PHCT) were confused as to their job. *continued*

Table 3.2:   Continued

Problems (continued)	• Social workers felt isolated from managerial and colleague support in district teams, and did not receive support that had been promised (such as with extra workload).
	• Social workers felt too thinly spread between GP practices.
	• Social workers had high workloads with little support.
	• Social workers felt most referrals were 'inappropriate', i.e. for benefits or housing enquiries.
	• Multi-disciplinary assessments were not noticeably more prompt or better quality.
Sustainability and transferability	• The lack of care management meant that these attachments were 'additional' to mainstream social services. Once project funding ran out it would have to be replaced by new additional funding.
	• There were no plans to transfer the project to other areas.

Source: Claridge B and Rivers P (1997) *Evaluation of Social Workers Attached to GP Practices: Report to Southern Derbyshire Health Authority.* University of Derby School of Health and Community Studies.

Table 3.3:   Practice-based social workers in South Worcestershire

Description	• Social workers based in six GP surgeries in South Worcestershire, employed by the social services department.
Funding	• Some posts were funded through practice underspends and social services grants, others through mainstream SSD funding.
Management of project	• Diverse; no central project team overseeing all six projects.
Supervision and management of care managers	• Social workers supervised by their team leaders (in the relevant area team).

continued

Table 3.3: Continued

Day-to-day running	• Social workers based in practice took referrals from GP practice, community nurses, patients and their families for all patients registered with the surgery. They carried out a full range of care management tasks, as well as providing welfare benefits advice and counselling. Patients with learning disabilities, mental health problems and childcare problems were referred to specialist social work teams.
Key findings	• There was no significant difference in the amount spent on services between the practice-based social workers and those based in area teams.
	• Primary care professionals and social workers perceived better 'early intervention' work and prevention of crises.
	• Patients and primary care professionals experienced better continuity of care.
	• Quicker referrals and response times.
	• Greater job satisfaction for GPs.
	• Easier access to social care for patients.
	• Improved interprofessional work and co-operation (particularly with community nurses).
Problems	• Benefits varied according to GPs – some showed less commitment and were less willing to refer patients than others.
	• Administrative support for the social workers proved problematic (because based in SSD).
	• Initial problems because of lack of preparation; GPs and social workers were unaware of the different working patterns and responsibilities of the other side. Some of these were resolved as the project progressed.
	• Problems for area SSD teams because practice-based social workers were not available to cover duty rosters or absences in team.
	• Some social workers felt isolated from their team and did not feel they received enough supervision.
	• Relations with specialist SSD teams were difficult.

continued

Table 3.3: Continued

Problems (continued)	• SSD was willing to adapt procedures to enable practice-based social workers to function, but this was not generally appreciated by primary care professionals.
Sustainability and transferability	• Concern was raised about the long-term funding of the project: it was felt that they should be SSD rather than NHS funded. However, there was support for extending the scheme from both the local and health authority. The situation was complicated by the restructuring of the local authority.

Source: Cumella S and Le Mesurier N (1997) *Social Work in Practice: an evaluation of social work in GP practices in South Worcestershire.* The Martley Press, Worcester.

Table 3.4: Castlefields Social Care Project

Description	• Unqualified social worker, based in Castlefields (Runcorn) practice, who acted for practice patients over 65.
Funding	• Jointly funded by SSD, health authority and Total Purchasing Pilot Practice.
Management of project	• The project emerged from earlier collaborative projects (such as the development of a practice agreement with social services) and was overseen by both the practice management (including a lead GP) and SSD.
Supervision and management of care managers	• The project worker was supervised by the team leader in the area team, and received support from a qualified social worker who carried out care management tasks for the practice patients that the project worker could not do herself.
Day-to-day running	• Project worker worked half-time in practice, half-time in SSD area team. • Project worker dealt with referrals for all over-65 year olds registered at the practice.

continued

Table 3.4:   Continued

Key findings	• Primary care professionals experienced considerable benefits, including easier access to social services for patients.
	• Primary care professionals reported reduced delays and frustration and better understanding of SSD policies and procedures.
	• Patients appreciated continuity of care from named worker.
	• Improved communication between primary care professionals and SSD.
Problems	• Posed equity problems for SSD because improved access to social services could not be replicated across the county.
	• Project worker had a very heavy workload compared to colleagues in area team.
	• Primary care professionals and SSD management still held each other in 'mutual mistrust' and project worker could get caught up between differing objectives and approaches.
Sustainability and transferability	• It was not considered possible to transfer the project to cover the county.

Source: Abbott S (1997) *The Castlefields Social Care Project: an evaluation.* Research
Report 96/35 Health and Community Care Research Unit, University of Liverpool.

KEY BENEFITS AND DISADVANTAGES OF CO-LOCATION/ATTACHMENT SCHEMES IN A PRIMARY CARE SETTING

Local and health authority managers' perspectives

There is some evidence that enabling patients to have easier access
to a social care worker (one of the main benefits of these schemes
for patients) results in earlier, lower cost interventions being used,

fewer emergency admissions to hospitals and less use of expensive residential and nursing home care.

However, it is notoriously difficult to quantify this evidence, because it is based on workers' assumptions and perceptions of what *might have happened* in alternative situations. It is, therefore, difficult to confirm that schemes of this type offer substantial cost-effectiveness savings. However, there is evidence that these schemes do not result in substantial *increases* in expenditure on either NHS or SSD care for patients, and that the improvements in procedures benefit both patients and health and social care workers. It does appear that these schemes offer at least the same *level* (and possibly better) of services at no increased *cost,* and therefore might offer a more *effective* and *efficient* way of delivering services.

Nevertheless, it does appear that these schemes offer better benefits to primary care professionals than social care workers, and may require more upheaval in working practices for social services managers than their health authority or primary care counterparts. This should be taken into account when planning or funding any co-location/attachment scheme.

- **These schemes may result in lower use of hospital beds and less use of institutional care.**
- **They offer a more effective way of accessing services for patients without a significant increase in the cost of services.**
- **The costs to social services appear to be greater (and the benefits lower) than for primary care professionals.**

Primary care professionals' perspectives

It is clear that the most significant benefits of these schemes are felt by primary care professionals. They gain an extra member of their team, with complementary skills, for the benefit of their patients. They gain quicker access to social services by having the worker on-site and through the worker to the rest of social services. They experience reduced frustration and delays because of improvements in referral and follow-up procedures and times. They often report improved job satisfaction because of these benefits.

Some schemes reported improved health outcomes for their patients, and fewer 'inappropriate' GP visits. However, these benefits were reported by primary care professionals and none of the evaluations substantiated these claims with quantifiable evidence. Nevertheless, a perceived reduction in patients attending busy surgeries with 'social' rather than 'health' problems was a significant factor in the improved job satisfaction reported by health workers, particulary GPs.

Community nurses were often surprised at how much they benefited from the schemes, given that they were rarely involved from the outset. They reported improved communication, reduced delays in referrals and better feedback. Some schemes also reported improvements in joint assessments, although these were more likely to happen when community nurses were significantly involved in the scheme from the beginning.

The only drawbacks for primary care professionals appeared to be that the social care workers could not always provide them with the level of service they expected and were limited to working according to SSD hours and procedures. This is likely to be a feature of unrealistic expectations at the outset of the scheme rather than a long-term problem. Not all primary care professionals benefited equally; some GPs were less interested, and so less involved, than others, and the importance of involving community nurses was not always appreciated at the beginning of schemes.

- **Reduction in delays and frustration for the PHCT arise from improved communication, more effective working practices and better interprofessional understanding.**
- **The involvement of community nursing staff is particularly beneficial.**
- **Schemes may lead to a reduction in inappropriate GP consultations.**
- **Schemes cannot improve the social care services available to patients, or overcome budgetary limitations.**

Social care workers' perspectives

Some schemes did result in improved job satisfaction for social care workers. This was due to the improved interprofessional working and the increased sense of autonomy experienced by outposted or attached workers, as compared to their colleagues in the area teams.

However, there were some significant drawbacks for social care workers in these schemes. Many of them reported professional isolation, sometimes because they received inadequate supervisory support from their area teams, sometimes because not all primary care professionals were necessarily committed to or aware of their role. Social care workers reported being 'caught in the middle' of disputes between the NHS and SSD, particularly if their local authority managers were less than committed to the schemes. They were at the mercy of both unrealistic expectations from health workers, and mistrust and lack of support from their social services colleagues.

Social care workers also reported that the majority of 'compromises' in procedures and working practices had been made by them, and were sometimes unacknowledged or unappreciated by their healthcare colleagues. Sometimes the tasks of 'networking' and informing health colleagues about their role was rewarding for social care workers, but it did increase their workload. Some social care workers found it difficult to work in a medically dominated environment, where issues such as anti-discriminatory practice and user involvement were considered much less important than they are in social care practice.

- **Some social care workers reported increased job satisfaction due to interprofessional working and greater autonomy.**
- **However, most reported an increase in professional isolation.**
- **Greater changes in working practices, sometimes compromising professional ethics, were required of social care than healthcare workers.**

- **The extra work put into networking and adjusting working practices was not always understood or acknowledged by healthcare workers.**

Patients' perspectives

The greatest benefits reported by patients in these schemes were the streamlining and simplification of procedures, and easier access to social care services. The easier access was two-fold: firstly, patients usually gained access to a named worker and avoided the bureaucracy associated with gaining access to mainstream SSD workers; secondly, patients preferred to access social care through the non-stigmatising route of primary care.

However, there was no evidence that patients received services that met their needs better than they would have done through mainstream SSD workers, either in terms of quantity (hours of services or money spent on services) or quality (services designed around their needs, rather than what was available and convenient for service providers). Extra services provided under some schemes (such as counselling, welfare rights or assistance with housing problems) were not considered to be part of their 'core' work by social care workers, even though they were valued highly by both patients and primary care professionals.

The drawbacks of these schemes for patients reflect the lack of patient involvement in establishing co-location projects. Patients were rarely given the chance to articulate what changes or improvements to services and service delivery they would like to see from their primary healthcare team, and schemes were usually designed and managed by the organisations funding them (usually the local authority and GP practice, sometimes the health authority), with no patient involvement.

- **Patients experienced easier access to services.**
- **There was no improvement in the services themselves.**

- **Lack of patient consultation or involvement in the design and management of schemes meant that their preferences were often not addressed.**

CREATING SUCCESSFUL SCHEMES

However successful co-location schemes have proved in primary care (in terms of improving interprofessional communication, improving access to social care for patients, reducing delays in referrals and service delivery, etc.), it has proved difficult to sustain and transfer these schemes widely.

- First, *many schemes have been set up using 'specialised' project finance* (such as special transitional grant money, total purchasing money, joint finance). When this funding runs out, it can be difficult to find the money to sustain projects, particularly as new budgetary pressures and priorities will have developed in the meantime. The end of GP fundholding and total purchasing may add to this problem and emphasises the need for secure, mainstream, long-term funding for such projects. The use of pooled budgets under the *Partnership in Action* flexibilities may go some way towards addressing this issue.
- Secondly, *most schemes that failed to be sustainable failed because the participants did not acknowledge the particular barriers to collaboration in primary care*, and thus failed to plan and implement ways of overcoming those barriers. Projects which had over-ambitious goals or which did not secure the commitment and co-operation of key participants, often failed.
- Finally, as was seen in the above section, *the benefits and disadvantages of co-location schemes tended to be disproportionately distributed*. Social services experienced more disadvantages (for example, isolation of social care workers, disruption and changes to procedures, provision of extra supervision and support) whilst primary care professionals experienced more

benefits (for example, quicker and easier access to social care, reduced frustration, greater job satisfaction). It is therefore not surprising that most SSDs proved unwilling to provide the funding necessary to sustain or transfer schemes.

However, there are elements that distinguish successful schemes. These elements, as they apply to the different groups involved, are discussed below.

Success factors for health and local authority managers

Successful schemes were characterised by careful planning and joint commitment from managers, who were usually the people with the power to put in place the support structures necessary for good day-to-day functioning of co-location/attachment schemes in primary care settings. Most importantly, there have to be clear benefits for both sides. The disproportionate burden borne by social services needs to be acknowledged and compensated for, for example by co-funding of posts or new services, or the provision of extra administrative support.

Organisational issues need to be sorted out, ideally before the scheme starts, so that frontline workers are able to start work straight away with sufficient support. Many schemes reported a lengthy delay in seeing benefits because issues such as administrative support, the role and responsibilities of the social care worker, the involvement of GPs and community nurses, and the relationship between the attached social care worker and mainstream SSD activity had not been fully negotiated at the start.

A development period, sometimes with an outside development worker, at the outset of schemes often proved invaluable in educating both sides about each others' roles and responsibilities, and in involving patients in the design and running of schemes. Although an additional investment, it often avoided the 'wasted' time at the beginning of projects while participants found their feet and negotiated their roles, and was useful in removing the barriers to collaboration.

Finally, a steering group of key managers from health and local authorities who were committed to the project often facilitated the negotiations and changes of direction that were evident in all the schemes. Successful schemes were often distinguished from those that failed because they managed to adapt to changing circumstances and adopted an incremental approach to development. This is much easier to achieve with the support and commitment of key budget holders in both health and local authorities. Even if the projects did not prove sustainable, the joint working achieved in such steering groups facilitated other projects and helped to break down inter-organisational barriers to collaboration.

- **Schemes need to be carefully planned.**
- **Commitment from both sides, at appropriate management levels is required.**
- **There need to be benefits for both sides.**
- **Schemes need to be adaptable, and this is aided by ongoing support from key managers.**

Success factors for primary care professionals

As was seen above, primary care professionals usually derive significant benefits from co-location/attachment schemes, but may lose these benefits because the projects are not sustainable. There are steps that can be taken by primary care professionals to aid the success of such projects.

First, the commitment and co-operation of all primary care professionals involved need to be secured. Efforts need to be made by all GPs, not just one 'enthusiastic' partner, to ensure that communication between health and social care workers is improved, including making an effort to be available for project meetings and referral discussions. Similarly, the involvement and commitment of community nurses need to be ensured; they will often be of vital importance in developing collaborative joint working, so need to be involved in the planning and implementation of the project.

Second, it is unfair for primary care professionals to expect social care workers to radically change their way of working without being willing to do the same. There is little point arguing that social care workers are bureaucratic and never available, if community nurses and GPs are unwilling to share information with social care workers in a convenient way. Many schemes found that 'insurmountable differences' in ways of working were actually quite easily overcome following sensible discussion and negotiation; for example, by community nurses being available for a regular session during the social care workers' office hours, or by setting up a short weekly 'progress report' meeting to facilitate the sharing of information.

Finally, primary care professionals need to be realistic about what social care workers can achieve. They need to be aware of SSD procedures and criteria, and that social care workers need to work with professional supervision. They also need to be aware of issues such as service charges, the importance of anti-discriminatory practice and user involvement, all of which mean that social care workers cannot just 'prescribe' services as though they were medicines.

- **Commitment is needed from all primary care professionals involved.**
- **Primary care professionals need to be adaptable and willing to make changes in working practices.**
- **An awareness of the constraints facing social care workers, and being realistic about what schemes can achieve, will help ensure that schemes are sustainable.**

Success factors for social care workers

Much of the onus for making a success of a co-location/attachment project in primary care falls on the social care workers' shoulders.

They need to be able to relish challenges, and be adaptable and confident enough that their professional values will survive working in a medically dominated setting. They also need to be able to function with a higher degree of autonomy and less peer support than their colleagues in mainstream social services teams.

Some role limitations and procedures which conventionally circumscribe mainstream social services activities may need to be reviewed. Attached or co-located workers will need to accept that they will not work in the same way as their colleagues in area teams; they will often find themselves acting as a liaison between patients/primary care professionals and the wider local authority, and carrying out tasks that would, in their area teams, be passed on to others.

They will also need to ensure that their primary care colleagues are aware of SSD responsibilities and procedures, and be able to adapt their working practices (such as office hours, forms, etc.) to fit in with the primary healthcare team. They will need to be prepared for the professional isolation that they are likely to experience.

- **Social care workers need to be well trained, experienced and professionally confident.**
- **They need to be adaptable and be willing to change accepted working practices.**
- **They need good networking and communication skills.**

Success factors for patients

Unfortunately, unless they are given an opportunity through participating in the development phase of a project, there is very little patients can do to ensure the success of an attachment or co-location scheme in a primary care setting, other than by singing its praises to a researcher if the scheme is evaluated.

ISSUES FOR FRONTLINE PRIMARY CARE/SSD COLLABORATION UNDER *THE NEW NHS*

What key lessons can be learnt from attachment/co-location schemes for primary care/social services collaboration in *The New NHS*? Does the lack of sustainability or transferability among many of even the 'successful' schemes signal the death knell for collaboration?

Firstly, there are ways of capturing some of the benefits of co-location/attachment schemes without having to set up expensive schemes to cover all the practices within a PCG/T.

- Practices can negotiate a practice agreement with social services (PASS), which can include such details as a named worker for referrals, agreed response times, ways of keeping each other informed of the progress of referrals, and so on.
- If PCG/Ts are formed as co-terminously as possible with social services boundaries, it may be possible to negotiate practice 'aligned' social care workers, who, while working within area teams, are the named worker for a group of practices, thus enabling easier interprofessional communication and collaboration. For example, this is currently being negotiated in Greenwich, where it proved financially impossible to roll out a very successful co-location project into more primary care settings.
- Liaison workers (usually jointly funded by health authorities and social services) have been shown to improve communication between primary care professionals and the SSD without substantial service reorganisation being necessary.[18]

Second, the following lessons for successful collaboration drawn from co-location/attachment schemes are equally applicable to collaboration between PCG/Ts and social services.

- The commitment of key managers and budget holders in both organisations is necessary for sustainable collaboration.
- Collaboration needs to have benefits for *both* parties involved; the costs of collaboration should not be borne unequally by one side.
- Participants need to have realistic, achievable goals.
- The roles and responsibilities of participants need to be clearly understood at the outset.
- It is particularly important to ensure that community nurses are fully involved.
- The barriers to interorganisational and interprofessional collaboration need to be acknowledged and addressed.
- Patients need to be involved to ensure that plans reflect their needs and priorities. This is unlikely to happen without sufficient development support.

REFERENCES

1 Lewis J and Glennerster H (1996) *Implementing the New Community Care.* Open University Press, Buckingham.

2 Davis A, Ellis K and Rummery K (1997) *Accessing Assessment: the perspectives of practitioners, disabled people and carers.* Policy Press, Bristol.

3 Rummery K and Glendinning C (1999) Negotiating needs, access and gatekeeping: developments in health and community care policies in the UK and the rights of disabled and older citizens. *Critical Social Policy.* **19**(3): 335–51.

4 Audit Commission (1996) *Balancing the Care Equation: progress with community care.* The Stationery Office, London.

5 Beattie A (1994) Health alliances or dangerous liaisons? The challenges of working together in health promotion. In: A Leathard (ed) *Going Interprofessional: working together for health and welfare.* Routledge, London.

6 Lymbery M (1998) Social work in general practice: dilemmas and solutions. *Journal of Interprofessional Care.* **12**(2): 199–208.

7   Audit Commission (1992) *Community Care: managing the cascade of change.* HMSO, London.

8   DETR (1998) *Modernising Local Government: improving local services through best value.* DETR, London.

9   Her Majesty's Government (1998) *Modern Local Government: in touch with the people,* Cm 4014. The Stationery Office, London.

10 Hudson B (1999) Decentralisation and primary care groups: a paradigm shift for the National Health Service in England? *Policy and Politics.* **27**(2): 159–72.

11 Department of Health (1997) *The New NHS: modern, dependable,* Cm 3807. The Stationery Office, London.

12 Department of Health (1998) *Modernising Health and Social Services: national priorities guidance* 1999/00–2001/02. The Stationery Office, London.

13 Poulton BC and West MA (1994) Primary health care team effectiveness: developing a constituency approach. *Health and Social Care in the Community.* **2**: 77–84.

14 Lewis J (1997) *Independent Contractors: GPs and the GP contract in the post-war period.* NPCRDC Debates in Primary Care 1, Manchester.

15 Klein R (1983) *The Politics of the National Health Service.* Longman, London.

16 Glendinning C (1998) From general practice to primary care: developments in primary health services 1990–98. In: E Brunsdon, H Dean and R Woods (eds) *Social Policy Review 10.* Social Policy Association, London.

17 Barnes M (1999) Users as citizens: collective action and the local governance of welfare. *Social Policy and Administration.* **33**(1): 73–90.

18 Tucker C and Brown L (1997) *Evaluating Different Models for Jointly Commissioning Community Care.* Wiltshire Social Services and University of Bath Research and Development Partnership Report 4, Bath.

FURTHER READING

Evaluated co-location or attachment projects

McNally D and Mercer N (1996) *Social Workers Attached to Practices: project report*. Knowsley Metropolitan Borough and Knowsley Health, Knowsley.

Pithouse A and Butler I (1994) Social work attachment in a group practice: a case study in success? *Research, Policy and Planning*. **12**(1): 16–20.

Ross F and Tissier J (1997) The care management interface with general practice: a case study. *Health and Social Care in the Community*. **5**(3): 153–61.

Stannard J (1996) *City Attached Care Manager Pilot: final report*. Hampshire Social Services, Winchester.

Tucker C and Brown L (1997) *Evaluating Different Models for Jointly Commissioning Community Care*. Wiltshire Social Services and University of Bath Research and Development Partnership Report 4, Bath.

Interprofessional working

Meads G (ed) (1997) *Health and Social Services in Primary Care: an effective combination?* Pearson Professional, London.

Øvretveit J *et al.* (eds) (1997) *Interprofessional Working for Health and Social Care*. Macmillan, Basingstoke.

Owens P *et al.* (eds) (1995) *Interprofessional Issues in Community and Primary Healthcare*. Macmillan, Basingstoke.

Vanclay L (1996) *Sustaining Collaboration Between General Practitioners and Social Workers*. CAIPE, London.

4

How do we know when we've got there? Evaluating frontline collaboration projects

Frontline collaboration projects of the type described in the previous chapter tend to be pilot projects, often with specific funding and a designated running period, although many of them have become part of mainstream services at the end of their 'pilot' period. Important questions for any manager or practitioner involved in such a project are whether or not it has achieved its goals, and whether or not it can be rolled out or transferred to other locations. This chapter will give an outline of the key factors to be considered in planning an evaluation of a frontline collaboration project, drawing on experiences of researchers involved in evaluating projects such as those described in the previous chapter.

FACTORS TO CONSIDER IN PLANNING AN EVALUATION

Evaluations that are not planned properly are likely to be inefficient and gather data that does not necessarily offer useful conclusions as to whether or not the project was a success. Ideally, the following issues need to have been addressed *before* the project has started.

Timing

Planning of any evaluation generally needs to take place *at the same time* as the planning of the project. Although it is possible to design an evaluation after a project is up and running, this does entail the risk that the evaluation will be less effective.

Purpose

The evidence presented in the previous chapter pointed out how crucial it is that projects have clear, realistic and achievable aims that are shared by the participants. Exactly the same can be said of evaluations. Why is the project being evaluated? What are the key questions that need answering?

It is crucial to the success of any evaluation that the questions it is attempting to answer are:

- the right questions (i.e. they are important to the managers, practitioners and other participants in the project), and
- answerable (i.e. it is feasible to answer them within the constraints of the project, and that the results are measurable in some way), and

- relevant to the stated aims of the project (i.e. that the outcomes being measured are those that the project was attempting to achieve).

The aims of the evaluation will dictate what type of evaluation is carried out, by whom, and using what data. If the aims of the evaluation are not clearly set out in the beginning, there is a danger that a great deal of useless data will be collected, and that data which would have been useful will have been left out.

It is also important for the commissioners of evaluations to be as honest as possible about the purposes of the evaluation, particularly if the project's viability depends on the outcome of the evaluation.[1,2]

Table 4.1: Aims of evaluation of Castlefields Social Care Project

- To gather the views of all relevant health and social services staff on the past, present and future value of the project.
- To investigate response times at the Castlefields Social Care Project.
- To investigate the use of social care services by those accessing them via the social care project in comparison with other districts in Cheshire.
- To compare workload and mode of service delivery of the Castlefields social care manager with other social services care managers.

Source: Abbott S (1997) *The Castlefields Social Care Project: an evaluation.* Health and Community Care Research Unit, University of Liverpool.

Who should be consulted?

Anyone designing an evaluation should plan to consult those involved as widely as possible *before* they begin work on the design. Who needs to be consulted will vary according to the nature of the project, but the following list is a useful general guideline.

- *All stakeholders.* Anyone who is involved in the project will need to be consulted about the evaluation while it is still in its planning stage. This includes any workers in the project, managers

who are overseeing or funding the project, primary care professionals who may be affected by the project, patients and their
families.

- *Other interested parties.* Even if they are not directly involved in
  the project, it can be useful to consult more widely within the
  health and local authority, and with groups such as the Local
  Medical Committee and Community Health Council.
- *Anyone who will be affected by the evaluation.* If they are not
  included in either of the above categories, it is a good idea to
  consult with anyone who may be affected by the evaluation,
  particularly people whose co-operation will be needed for
  data collection (such as practice managers, receptionists, local
  authority workers).
- *Whoever will be carrying out the evaluation.* Although deciding
  who should do the evaluation is part of planning it (*see* p. 82),
  once that decision has been made they need to be involved in
  the consultation process as well as the evaluation itself.

However, it is important during the consultation process not to
lose sight of what the evaluation is for, nor end up with a long list
of unanswerable questions. It may be interesting to track the
health outcomes of a large group of patients, but it will not
necessarily reveal whether a particular project has been successful
in overcoming interprofessional barriers.

What kind of evaluation is needed?

The type of evaluation will depend not only on the *purpose* of
the evaluation (although this is the most important consideration)
but also on other factors such as *cost* and *time constraints*. The
NHSE (1997)[2] distinguishes between three different types of
evaluation.

- *Project monitoring.* This is where costs, inputs, outputs and the
  activity of a project are measured. This information comprises

the building blocks of evaluation rather than full evaluation itself. However, if funds and time are limited, carrying out thorough project monitoring is more useful and cost effective than carrying out a partial and flawed outcome evaluation.

• *Process evaluation.* This evaluates the development of a project, usually to assess whether or not it can be sustained or transferred to other areas. Its purpose is to identify and address any problems or barriers to success.

• *Outcome evaluation.* This is where the effectiveness of the project in meeting its aims is assessed. One dimension of outcome evaluation is *economic* evaluation, where the costs and benefits of a project are analysed.

These categories may be combined in practice. For example, one element of process evaluation often involves assessing *intermediate* outcomes, which are part of the process of achieving final outcomes. For example, an increase in the take-up of a particular service could be an intermediate outcome on the way towards an increase in the quality of life which that service is meant to deliver. One element of a successful (or failed) outcome can be an assessment of the *process* of the project. Neither process nor outcome evaluation is possible without the information that is gathered during project monitoring.

However, in deciding which type of evaluation to conduct, it can be helpful to think about the relationship between the aims of the project and what information is needed to assess whether those aims have been met. If the costs and benefits of practice-attached care managers are already known, then a *process* evaluation of one such project, to ascertain which elements worked and which were barriers to collaboration, may be more cost effective than attempting to track the outcomes for practitioners and patients. Similarly, if a project's aim is to show improved health gain and quicker response times, then it will be necessary to measure *outcomes* (compared to baseline data) to ascertain whether or not these have been achieved.

Who should carry out the evaluation?

This will depend on the purpose and type of evaluation planned, and cost and timing considerations. It is always advisable that the evaluation is *not* carried out by any of the stakeholders. It would be very difficult for anyone with a direct interest or involvement in the project to be able to gather and analyse data which may affect the future of the project.

However, it is not always easy to identify stakeholders. An outside 'independent' body, whether an academic unit or consultancy, may become a stakeholder through being involved in the project, for example through providing developmental or managerial support to the project.

Whoever carries out the evaluation, it is important that they have the skills and resources to do so. Again, this will depend on the type of evaluation needed, but could include:

- health economics expertise
- statistical skills
- interviewing and survey skills
- dissemination (presenting the findings to a range of audiences) expertise.

The following range of people are likely to be able to carry out evaluations:

- practitioners, perhaps from other practices/trusts/teams (but attention should be paid to whether their practice/trust/team is likely to be affected by the project, which would make them an indirect stakeholder)
- research officers in health and local authorities (again, attention should be paid to their potential stakeholder status)
- academics with expertise in primary/social care collaboration
- health/social service management consultancies.

MEASURING THE SUCCESS (AND FAILURE) OF A PROJECT

Once decisions have been taken about the aims of an evaluation and who should carry it out, it is time to think about the design and execution of an evaluation. This section will briefly discuss what needs to be taken into account when designing an evaluation, and some of the ways of measuring both processes and outcomes.

Designing the evaluation

The design of the evaluation should be based on both the project's aims and the objectives of the evaluation. Once these have been established, it is necessary to decide on the design and scope of the evaluation, and draw up an evaluation plan. The NHSE[2] recommend that an evaluation plan should contain the following:

- justification for the design and methods chosen
- specific data collection methods used
- sample size required
- sampling strategy
- setting for data collection
- methods of data analysis including any computer support needs.

The team which designed and carried out the evaluation of the Greenwich practice-based care management project described in the previous chapter (see Table 3.1) decided that their overarching aim for the evaluation was to identify the added value of having a practice-based care manager over other models of joint working between primary health and social care in the locality. They then linked the objectives of the project to the evaluation design as shown in Table 4.2.

Table 4.2: Evaluation design of Greenwich practice-based care management project

Objective	How measured?
Establish two pilot GP practices where a care manager would be based	This objective was overachieved by the end of the developmental year, at which point three care managers were working with nine GP practices
Ensure that the practice-based care manager is a permanent member of the primary care team	• Interviews with staff, care managers, GPs, practice nurses, support workers, practice managers and receptionists. • Participant observation through regular visits to each practice. • Attending practice meetings.
Develop a more effective 'seamless' way of managing the joint health and social care needs of the practice patients	• Attending practice meetings. • Tracking referrals via computer database.
To provide the most appropriate care for patients	• Interview with patients. • Observation at practice meetings.
To test the costs and benefits of incorporating social care into primary healthcare	• Monitoring budget information (spend per client) by specially designated software. • Monitoring case loads and tracking referrals. • Monitoring time spent on project by staff (GPs, senior care managers, district nurses).
Develop systems for purchasing care and support across both health and social services	• Regular liaison with project staff during data collection visits to practices. • Tracking budget data.

Source: Hodgson CR (1997) *It's All Good Practice: evaluating practice-based care management in Greenwich.* South East Institute of Public Health.

This evaluation included a mixture of qualitative and quantitative, process and outcome measures, while avoiding collecting data that would give little insight into how the project was achieving its objectives. However, it was a time-consuming and fairly large-scale evaluation, which took place over the three years of the life of the project.

Measuring process

Evaluating the process of a project can give managers valuable information about the *progress* a project makes towards achieving its objectives. This type of information can be useful when thinking about whether and how to transfer or 'roll out' a successful project. It enables the participants to understand *how* they achieved their objectives.

As in any evaluation, the information needed to assess the process of a project comes from *project monitoring*. This consists of data on the *costs, inputs, activities* and *outputs* of the project. The NHSE suggest that the following questions may be useful guidelines for process evaluations:

* which aspects of the project are being successfully implemented/ which have not been successfully realised?
* what unanticipated problems or effects have been identified?
* what factors are facilitating successful implementation/what factors are proving barriers to change?
* how easy is it to implement the project?
* how acceptable is the project to different stakeholders?

The team which carried out the evaluation of the social workers attached to GP practices project in South Derbyshire were concerned with measuring the *process* of the project. The aims of that project and the evaluation methodology used are summarised in Table 4.3.

As can be seen from the methodology, the intention of this evaluation was not to measure the achievement of the project's goals, but to assess *progress towards* those goals. For this reason,

Table 4.3: Evaluation methodology

Project aims	Evaluation methodology
• Obtain greater levels of integrated working. • Improve access to services for patients. • Improve communication and joint working between GP practices and social services.	• Monitoring forms filled in by social workers. • Focus groups with stakeholders. • Unstructured and semi-structured interviews with stakeholders (including two patients).

Source: Claridge B and Rivers P (1997) *Evaluation of Social Workers Attached to GP Practices: Report to South Derbyshire Health Authority.* School of Health and Community Studies, University of Derby.

there was no effort made to gather data which could compare the project with conventional methods of service delivery. The quantitative data which was collected on the monitoring forms only compared the two social workers in different practices, and it did not provide any comparison with mainstream social workers.

This evaluation was not extensive, and was only commissioned 18 months after the start of the project. It was, therefore, nearly impossible for the evaluators to provide any reasonable information on outcomes of the project as they had not been able to gather 'baseline' data at the start. However, this evaluation did provide information on the difficulties and barriers to collaborative working in the practices.

Measuring outcomes

Outcome evaluation is designed to show whether or not a project has achieved its aims. It tends to be more comprehensive and costly than process evaluation, and hence may not always be the most cost-effective way of assessing a project. Because of the costs of this type of evaluation, it is vital that the measures chosen to assess outcomes are useful and feasible.

A great deal of attention in health services research is paid to ways of measuring *health status* and *outcomes*. There are several well-known and validated ways of doing this, such as the Nottingham Health Profile and the health status measure SF-36.[3] However, such measures are only of use if one of the project's aims was specifically to improve the health status of its patients. This has not tended to be a feature of frontline collaboration projects, whose aims have generally been more concerned with improving *access* to care for patients and practitioners.

Several academics have argued that it is impossible to construct a universal measure of *social care outcomes*, although this is being attempted by researchers working in the Outcomes of Social Care for Adults programme funded by the Department of Health. At present there are few validated ways of measuring social care outcomes.

However, the Greenwich, Castlefields and South Worcestershire teams of evaluators did make some attempt to measure the outcomes of the projects concerned. The methodology used by the South Worcestershire team, as well as the aims of the evaluation, are summarised in Table 4.4.

As can be seen, to carry out a full-scale outcome evaluation, using validated qualitative and quantitative measures, is a big undertaking. Nevertheless, it is the only way to reliably assess a project's performance against its objectives.

An important element of measuring outcomes is often a *cost-benefit analysis*. When designing this type of evaluation, it is important to bear in mind that *costs* include not only direct costs, but *opportunity costs* (the cost of activities foregone in favour of the project) and *marginal costs* (the extra costs incurred due to new activities in the project). Any cost-benefit analysis will only be of use if there is reliable *baseline data* from which to work. It is therefore necessary to consider what sort of cost-benefit analysis may form a feasible part of the evaluation.

Table 4.4: Evaluation of social workers in GP practices project, South Worcestershire

Evaluation aims	Methodology
• To evaluate the resource effectiveness of integrated health and social care in primary care teams. • To identify good practice in establishing integrated health and social care schemes in primary care. • To identify good practice in the management of major transition points for disabled people (the onset of disability, discharge from hospital, and assessment for institutional care). • To identify the organisational implications for health and social services of an extension of practice-based social work.	• Quasi-experimental design comparing six practice-based social workers with six practices without practice-based social workers. • Contact survey of patients with social workers over a 14-day fieldwork period. • Resource effectiveness study, 128 patients interviewed, measuring degree of disability (OPCS Disability Survey), health status (SF-36), mental state (Hospital Anxiety and Depression Scale) and receipt of services (receipt of services questionnaire, developed by researchers). • Organisational impact study, semi-structured interviews with stakeholders. • Case studies from social workers' records. • National postal survey of social services departments and health authorities to ascertain incidence of practice-based social workers.

Source: Cumella S *et al.* (1996) *Social Work in Practice: an evaluation of the care management received by elderly people from social workers based in GP practices in South Worcestershire.* The Martley Press, Worcester.

REFERENCES

1 Usherwood T (1996) *Introduction to Project Management in Health Research: a guide for new researchers.* Open University Press, Buckingham.

2   NHSE (1997) *Personal Medical Services Pilots under the NHS (Primary Care) Act 1997: a guide to local evaluation.* NHSE, Leeds.

3   Bowling A (1991) *Measuring Health: a review of quality of life measurement.* Open University Press, Buckingham.

FURTHER READING

Berk RA and Rossi PH (1990) *Thinking About Programme Evaluation.* Sage, Newbury Park, CA.

Drummond MF *et al.* (1987) *Methods for the Economic Evaluation of Healthcare Programmes.* Oxford University Press, Oxford.

King J *et al.* (1988) *How to Assess Program Implementation.* Sage, Newbury Park, CA.

Nocon A and Qureshi H (1996) *Outcomes of Community Care for Users and Carers: a social services perspective.* Open University Press, Buckingham.

Philips C *et al.* (1994) *Evaluating Health and Social Care.* Macmillan, Basingstoke.

Wilkin D *et al.* (1992) *Measures of Need and Outcome for Primary Healthcare.* Oxford University Press, Oxford.

5

Working in partnership for older people: new possibilities?

The landscape of primary and social care has undergone radical change over the past few years; this is set to continue as *The New NHS, Modernising Social Services, Partnership in Action* and other key policies are implemented. There will be continuing pressure on GPs, community nurses, health authority managers and their counterparts in local authorities to focus on the changes within their own organisations to the detriment of working in partnership. As some of the evidence in Chapter 2 shows, internal management and structural issues are likely to dominate the formation and functioning of PCGs in the first few years; working in partnership with outside agencies may take some time to develop effectively unless there is a history of good working relations and a set of common goals. Conversely, social services departments do not have a great deal of experience in engaging with primary care, particularly around service commissioning, and are also likely to be preoccupied with their own organisational concerns as local authorities undergo their own changes.

However, it is worth remembering that the health and wellbeing of older people, particularly frail older people, is a key concern for all these organisations and professionals. Commissioning and delivering effective services which enable older people to live independent lives in the community requires, at the very least, the co-ordination of health and social care. Notwithstanding this common interest in promoting and developing the health and well-being of older people, central government policy is also increasingly focusing on partnerships between statutory services as a vehicle for achieving social and economic, as well as health, improvements for localities. As was discussed in Chapter 1, the pressures to work in partnership to commission and deliver services for older people are only likely to increase.

This chapter will discuss the pitfalls and opportunities for primary health and social care partnership working that are likely to develop over the next few years.

LOCAL AUTHORITIES AND OLDER PEOPLE

New ways of delivering services for older people

Over the last decade local authorities have moved away from directly providing a range of services (including leisure, transport and housing as well as social services) to commissioning services from a variety of independent and statutory providers. This trend is set to continue under current government policy, with the obligation to secure the 'best value' when commissioning services for older people.

While social services departments remain the key partners for PCGs when commissioning and delivering services for older people, changes in the structures of local authorities may mean that barriers between social services departments and other local authority departments are removed or become less significant than they have been. Some local authorities have already combined traditional functions in new ways, such as amalgamating social services and housing departments.[1] Hudson has argued[2] that this, plus the push towards regionalisation of local government, is likely to make partnerships with the NHS more, not less, difficult. One study of interagency working involving housing, health and social care found that commitment to partnerships at one level within each organisation were not necessarily shared by those at other levels, leading to confusion and difficulties in translating joint plans into action.[3] New initiatives, such as 'Better Government for Older People', which are focused on reducing interorganisational barriers and delivering services to older people in a more stream-lined 'one-stop-shop' way, will also have implications for joint working with primary care.

Notwithstanding the difficulties that are likely to be caused by the changes *within* local authorities, as was discussed in Chapter 1, there are now clear obligations upon them to work in partnership with the NHS. As PCGs move towards PCT status they will take over more of the health authority's responsibilities for com-missioning health services to older people, as well as providing primary and community health services. PCGs will find them-selves obliged to work in partnership with the wider local authority to commission and provide health and other services for older people.

Partnership obligations

Strategically, local authorities are under an obligation to liaise with the NHS in implementing health improvement programmes and are liable, jointly with their NHS partners, to sign up to joint investment plans. They will no longer be able to work within joint consultative committees, but the ways they work in partnership with the NHS, particularly PCG/Ts, will be closely monitored.

The experience of working strategically together to commission services has shown that it is facilitated by having identifiable 'pots' of money to develop services. Partnership grants (totalling nearly £650 million over three years) are available to help local authority social services develop joint services that foster older people's independence in the community. These are complemented by a new £100 million prevention grant to target low-level support at people deemed to be at risk of losing their independence and encourage health and social care services to move away from crisis-intervention towards prevention and rehabilitation, reducing the risk of admission to hospital or residential/nursing care.

Operationally, local authorities will also be monitored on their achievement of multi-disciplinary assessments for older people in the community. These are valued by health and social care commissioners and practitioners who welcome the opportunity to co-ordinate the delivery of services as effectively as possible. Perhaps more importantly they are also valued by older people and their families, who often find it easier to make their wishes known in a 'structured' meeting of the relevant primary health and social care practitioners,[4] and who benefit from a reduction in delays resulting from improved care planning and management at the frontline. Local authorities (and the NHS) will be monitored under health improvement programmes to ensure that they jointly develop services which are 'co-ordinated and easily accessible, linking services and using "one-stop shops" where appropriate'.[5]

The flexibilities offered in the *Partnership in Action* proposals (discussed in more detail below) could facilitate joint working between local authorities and PCG/Ts at both the strategic (service commissioning) and operational (service delivery) level.

THE NEW LANDSCAPE OF PRIMARY CARE

PCGs and PCTs: the option to provide and commission integrated care

The New NHS deliberately avoided being over-prescriptive about how PCGs might function, stressing that 'what counts is what works'. The different levels of PCG, with varying degrees of responsibility for service commissioning, could translate into as many different models nationally as there are PCGs, given that the structure, function and relationship with health authorities are a matter for local agreeement. PCGs will move towards PCT status at varying paces: some may not wish to develop in this direction at all, although they may not be able to avoid it indefinitely. However, for PCGs to operate as level 4 PCTs they must take on the responsibility for *both* commissioning *and* providing a range of primary, community and secondary health services. These trusts will be able to function with a great deal of freedom from the health authority, employing community health staff, running community hospitals and providing integrated primary healthcare. Although GPs may remain as independent contractors, it is likely that increasing numbers of them in PCTs will opt to be employees of the trust.

Having salaried GPs could offer trusts valuable new flexible ways of delivering and commissioning services for older people. As independent contractors GPs have to negotiate payment for any non-GMS activities: this includes the management responsibilities associated with acting on a PCT board, and the work involved in developing services in partnership with outside agencies such as local authorities. The evidence from successful joint commissioning sites suggests that it is important to have sufficient and dedicated managerial support to enable services to be developed in partnership. Under the possibilities opened up by the 1997 Primary Care Act it is now possible for GPs to opt for salaried status under a Personal Medical Services (PMS) based contract, with much greater local flexibility than the traditional GMS contract. PCTs could, by being able to set the terms and conditions of employment, support the full involvement of GPs in service development as well as the provision of healthcare for older people.

In order to attain trust status, PCGs will need to show that they are 'making an effective contribution and working within the health improvement programe set by the health authority *and partner organisations*' (Annex A in *The New NHS: modern, dependable*, emphasis added). PCTs are also required to have local authority representation on their governing bodies (in the case of PCGs this obligation is limited to social services representation) and this will offer opportunities to set an agenda for service commissioning in partnership with local authorities. PCTs will therefore have a combination of duties to provide *and* commission integrated health services, and may provide primary care professionals with a range of opportunities to work in partnership with other agencies in setting commissioning priorities. This makes the formation of PCTs a significant departure from previous attempts at involving primary care in service commissioning (such as fundholding, total purchasing and GP commissioning) in which primary care professionals (overwhelmingly GPs) largely developed services according to their own perceptions of the needs of their patients, and did not make significant progress towards either population-based needs assessment or developing commissioning priorities in partnership with other stakeholders.[6]

PCTs could potentially operate like US health maintenance organisations (HMOs), who take the responsibility for purchasing *and* providing integrated health and social care pathways for older people. Although they cannot 'compete' for the health insurance money of older people in the way that HMOs do, they could, if necessary using *Partnership in Action* flexibilities, take on the responsibility for commissioning integrated health and social care services for their older patients. However, not all PCTs will be ready (or willing) to take on such ambitious joint commissioning. Early indications suggest that issues such as clinical governance (particularly establishing clear mechanisms for the managerial and peer review of clinical activities) will be the preoccupation of many trusts in the initial stages. Nevertheless, the experience of successful joint commissioning shows that where NHS and local authority colleagues have to work together, they can overcome historical differences and develop a shared agenda fairly quickly. With imagination and a commitment to joint working, PCTs have an unprecedented opportunity to work with their social services counterparts to commission and provide truly integrated health and social care services for their older patients.

Partnership obligations

As PCGs develop and acquire increasing levels of responsibility and autonomy, so the opportunities to engage in collaborative activities with local authority services will increase. For example, PCGs are likely gradually to become involved in assessing needs and commissioning services for vulnerable older people and those with complex needs, as part of the Joint Investment Planning process, alongside local authority partners. However, it is only when PCGs take on board the full range of possibilities opened up by achieving trust status that they will be able to exploit some of the more innovative options for working in partnership with social services. The flexibilities offered in the *Partnership in Action* proposals offer the potential for PCTs and social services to develop services for older people which not only integrate primary and community health services, but involve a range of rehabilitative and social services as well.

Exploiting the possibilities: *Partnership in Action* flexibilities

The 1999 NHS Act will enable PCGs and PCTs to overcome some of the organisational and budgetary barriers that have hindered partnership working with social services in the past. The first pilot sites to use the *Partnership in Action* flexibilities are likely to 'go live' in April 2000. Although not confined to partnerships in services for older people, the flexibilities could offer the potential for innovative service development in this area. *Partnership in Action* offers social services and NHS organisations the opportunity to either pool budgets, designate a lead commissioner or integrate service provision across a range of services.

Pooled budgets

It will be possible for PCG/Ts and local authorities to put a proportion of their funds into a joint budget, in which the separate funding streams would become integrated and can be spent commissioning services on the 'margins' of traditional health and social care boundaries.

In Australia, this has been attempted with the integration of State and Federal budgets to break down the traditional barriers between acute and continuing hospital and community health services.[7] The Australian pilots showed that it was necessary to ringfence budgets for non-medical services, echoing concerns in the UK that acute sector provision could dominate when hospital and community health funding streams were integrated. In Northern Ireland health and social care budgets have effectively been pooled since the imposition of direct rule in 1972. It has been possible to commission services which enable frail older people to avoid residential or nursing home care, such as intensive integrated home care and community nursing services.

However, simply pooling budgets does not remove the thorny issue of service charges. The commissioning of integrated intensive home care and nursing services in Northern Ireland was facilitated by the lack of local authority service charges. PCG/Ts and social services in England will not be able to avoid tackling the problem of users being charged for social care services while health services remain free at the point of delivery, if they pool their budgets to commission services which operate at the 'margins' of health and social care for older people. The problem will be particularly acute for those PCG/Ts which are working in partnership with more than one local authority and which have different charging policies and procedures.

Lead commissioning

This option is where one organisation transfers its statutory responsibilities to the other, who then takes responsibility for commissioning both health *and* social care services. Unlike the pooled budgets option, where both organisations can contribute to commissioning, this option entails one organisation delegating responsibility to the other. The 1999 NHS Act will enable both the statutory responsibilities and the funding to be transferred both ways. For example, PCTs could delegate the commissioning of rehabilitation or nursing services for older people to social services, so as to make use of their greater experience in commissioning services from a range of independent and statutory providers. Conversely, PCTs could take on the responsibility for commissioning residential care for older people from social services.

Such arrangements are likely to be most successful where there is a considerable degree of trust between both organisations involved, which would imply a history of good partnership working. However, as the evidence in Chapter 2 showed, commissioning relationships between primary care and social services remain underdeveloped, so it may be that many of the first wave of PCTs will be ill-prepared for designating social services as lead commissioner for services for older people. It is likely that this flexibility will be particularly useful in relation to relatively specialised services, such as those for people with complex physical and/or learning disabilities, where primary care has historically had little commissioning experience.

However, as relationships develop between PCTs and local authorities, delegating the responsibility for commissioning services for older people to each other may be an option to explore in the future. The issue of service charges will need to be addressed: there is a danger if commissioning responsibility is transferred to local authorities that services previously provided free by the NHS could become liable to charges under local authorities. This may prove politically sensitive and difficult for older people and their families, particularly in the light of the recommendation of the Royal Commission on long-term care that all personal and nursing care should be provided for older people free of charge.[8]

Integrated providers

Under this option, one organisation can provide both health and social care to older people. Using this option would enable PCTs to provide elements of social care to their older patients (perhaps intensive home care services, or hospital-at-home schemes using integrated nursing and home care teams); alternatively social services could provide some community health services on behalf of PCTs. An integrated health and social care provider team could also include salaried GPs.

It is often the co-ordination of frontline health and social care delivery that causes older people and their families the most concern. Some projects have used short-term winter pressures money to commission integrated intensive home care and nursing support for older people who have thus avoided hospital admission. In Northern Ireland (as discussed above) the pooled health and social care budget has meant it has been possible to provide integrated intensive home care and nursing services to older people living in the community and thus remove or delay the need for residential and nursing home care. In Denmark, integrated care teams, comprising nurses, occupational therapists, home helps and other health and social care professionals, provide a 24-hour service to frail older people living in their own homes, following successful pilot schemes in the 1980s.[9] Use of this flexibility in England would also enable PCTs to employ trained home care nursing staff so that one person could provide both nursing and domestic home care services to frail older people in their own homes (although the issue of service charges would still need addressing).

WORKING IN PARTNERSHIP WITH OLDER PEOPLE

Throughout this paper we have chosen to focus on partnerships between managers and professionals in the commissioning and provision of health and social care services for older people. However, the importance of partnerships between older people themselves and primary health and social care commissioners and providers should not be underestimated.

As the evidence in Chapters 2 and 3 shows, primary care is relatively inexperienced in involving patients in the setting of commissioning priorities or improving frontline collaboration. It appears that unless there is dedicated funding and support for patient involvement, it is unlikely to develop significantly within primary care-led commissioning. This reflects the under-development of public participation in the NHS in general, which has only seemed to flourish in one-off, well-supported projects (such as citizens' juries) rather than forming an integral part of service development. Local authorities, with their strong local democratic links and accountability to local tax payers, have a somewhat stronger history of local involvement in service development, for example in the production of community care plans.[10]

The underdevelopment of older people's involvement in health services commissioning is exacerbated by the view of many primary care professionals, particularly GPs, that *they* are the right people to represent their patients' needs. However, it has been pointed out that this often reflects what professionals *think* their patients' priorities are, rather than being a reflection of older people's actual experiences and views.[11] The doctor–patient relationship, where GPs act in the best *medical* interests as advocates (and gatekeepers to specialist services for specific medical conditions) for *individual* patients, does not map easily onto a model of service development that needs to deliver a wide range of services for *groups* of patients.

Four strategies have been suggested for involving patients in the NHS:[11]

- direct participation, for example on PCG/T boards
- informed views, for example through patient surveys
- community development, for example in involving local communities in health action zones
- local scrutiny and accountability, for example through greater local democratic accountability, rather than just accountability through health authorities to the Department of Health.

However, the training of many primary care professionals has left them ill-prepared to engage in dialogues with patients about developing service priorities. Support would be needed to ensure that older people's involvement was meaningful without being over-threatening to the professional status of GPs and other primary and community health workers who commission and provide services in PCG/Ts. However, projects such as the Fife User Panels show this has been done successfully in social services[12] and could be translated into PCG/Ts. The experience of the two joint commissioning projects highlighted in Chapter 2 which *did* have significant user involvement shows that primary care professionals can rise to the challenge of engaging with older people and their families, and even welcome the opportunity to develop new partnerships in this way.

REFERENCES

1   Craig G and Manthorpe J (1998) Small is beautiful? Local government reorganisation and the role of social services departments. *Policy and Politics.* **26**(3): 189–207.

2   Hudson B (1999) Decentralisation and primary care groups: a paradigm shift for the National Health Service in England? *Policy and Politics.* **27**(2): 159–72.

3   Arblaster L, Conway J, Foreman A and Hawtin M (1996) *Asking the Impossible? Inter-agency working to address the housing, health and social care needs of people in ordinary housing.* Policy Press, Bristol.

4   Baldock J and Ungerson C (1994) *Becoming Consumers of Care.* Joseph Rowntree Foundation, York.

5   Department of Health (1998) *Modernising Social Services: promoting independence, improving protection, raising standards,* Cm 4169. The Stationery Office, London.

6   Devlin M and Smith J (1999) States of flux. *Health Service Journal.* **May 6**: 24–5.

7   Fine M (1998) Acute and continuing care for older people in Australia: contesting new balances of care. In: Glendinning C (ed) *Rights and Realities: comparing new developments in long-term care for older people.* Polity Press, Bristol.

8   Royal Commission (1998) *With Respect to Old Age,* Cm 4192-I. The Stationery Office, London.

9   Lund Pedersen L (1998) Health and social care for older people in Denmark: a public solution under threat? In: Glendinning C (ed) *Rights and Realities: comparing new developments in long-term care for older people.* The Polity Press, Bristol.

10 Bewley C and Glendinning C (1994) *Involving Disabled People in Community Care Planning.* Joseph Rowntree Foundation, York.

11 Barnes M and Evans M (1998) Who wants a say in the NHS? *Health Matters.* **34**: 6–7.

12 Barnes M and Bennett-Emslie G (1997) *If They Would Listen: an evaluation of the Fife User Panels.* Age Concern Scotland, Edinburgh.

Index